My Dementia Defense

Also by Don Nicholson:
Ocular Pathology Update
Pediatric Ocular Tumors

My Dementia Defense

DON NICHOLSON

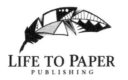

LIFE TO PAPER
PUBLISHING

First Edition 2024

Paperback ISBN: 978-1-990700-27-9
eBook ISBN: 978-1-990700-36-1

Library of Congress Control Number: 2024904662

Title page art © apratim/Adobe Stock

Printed in the U.S.A.
1 2 3 4 5 6 7 8 9 10

Life to Paper Publishing Inc.
Toronto | Miami

www.lifetopaper.com

LIFE TO PAPER
PUBLISHING

To you, the reader.

Gracias a la vida que me ha dado tanto.
Violeta Parra, 1966

There is a crack in everything.
That's how the light gets in.
Leonard Cohen, 1992

Gifts and Luck
All received,
Most well used.
Don Nicholson, 2023

Contents

Illustrations

Preface

In 2014, when I was almost 74, I began to lose words in daily conversation, and my memory wasn't as clear as I thought it should be. Helping care for my father's Alzheimer disease on my monthly visits to Memphis during the last 10 years of his life sensitized me to dementia.

Dr. Clinton Wright, head of geriatric memory at the University of Miami School of Medicine, put me through an exhaustive evaluation. Two days of psychological testing, a half-day social worker interview for me, two hours for Magda, laboratory tests, and neuroradiological studies. After he had thoroughly reviewed all the results, Dr. Wright[1] sat with the two of us. He was in his mid-forties with light brown hair and an intense expression.

"Dr. Nicholson, I'm afraid that the tests show that you do have Alzheimer disease. Here is a prescription for donepezil, which we believe slows progression. You should return to repeat the examinations in a year."

Huddling under the umbrella on our walk to the parking lot, Magda looked up at me. "Doesn't sound good, does it?" I smiled and vowed, "I'm going to be the Michael J. Fox of

---

1. Dr. Wright was promoted to Associate Director for the National Institute of Neurological Disorders and Stroke at the NIH. https://www.ninds.nih.gov/about-ninds/who-we-are/staff-directory/clinton-wright.

Alzheimer disease." After a few months trying to teach Magda to use Quicken to manage our family finances, we both gave up. I returned to denial, my original dementia defense.

Two years later we attended a book reading by an Alzheimer specialist and met the author, Dr. Marc Agronin, a well-known geriatric neuropsychiatrist at the Miami Jewish Health System. We made an appointment to see Dr. Agronin in four months.

He greeted us in his office with a broad smile and outstretched hand. He was medium size, of slim, athletic build. His face broadcast intelligence. He listened patiently to my story.

"We need a PET scan and to repeat the blood tests and psychological studies," he explained. "It's been two years since your tests by Dr. Wright, which I have reviewed. We should be able to determine whether there has been any progression."

The following week, his psychologist served a lob into my court of suicide. In retrospect, I should have slammed it back to her baseline as an "I have never thought about suicide" return. Instead, I hemmed, hawed, and lamely admitted that I didn't think that suicide was in all cases a bad idea. She turned in her chair and hit the panic button, a quick telephone call.

"Dr. Agronin would like to see you now," she stuttered, looking toward her office door.

"Can't we finish the tests first?" I asked.

"He-e wants to see you n-now."

An orderly walked me to a chair outside the doctor's office. I sat squirming while the orderly stood at paunchy attention.

I went inside. Dr. Agronin asked me about suicide for 30 minutes with rapid-fire questions, obviously well-practiced. He thought a moment, decided that I was not a suicide risk, and looked up. "You may finish the testing now."

While taking psychological tests for Alzheimer disease, do not let the word "suicide" even whiz through your amygdala, much less touch your tongue.

After the second day's testing, Magda and I sat in the doctor's office. "The test results actually show some improvement since the first set two years ago," Dr. Agronin said with a genuine smile, "Rather than Alzheimer disease, I think you have mild cognitive impairment, which may progress more slowly and have a better outcome."

When we were outside, Magda turned to me: "I'm glad Dr. Wright was wrong."

"Alzheimer Disease versus cognitive impairment," I replied. "You might be right. Or maybe Dr. Agronin just tried to use a less threatening term."

It took five years for me to realize that our relief that day was premature.

During the COVID-19 pandemic lockdown in 2020 I began writing a memoir for my grandchildren, *Notes for My Grandchildren*. Within a year, my sloppy keyboard writing showed that my memory had slipped further. My hunt-and-peck required the simultaneous coordination of thought, touch, and sight. If I had learned to type, thought and sight would have been sufficient, and I might have fooled myself a while longer.

"Mild" was the key word in Dr. Agronin's revised diagnosis. A short, simple, reassuring word that, unfortunately, may apply for only a brief time. I had dropped from mild toward moderate cognitive impairment. Instead of a few random comments jotted for future generations, my memoir became a lifeline, a map to keep me on my Michael J. Fox–inspired track.

I gave Magda a copy of the essential dementia caregiver guide, *The 36-Hour Day*, with the inscription:

"To Sarita with Love –
A gift I wish I never had to give you.
I'll love you forever, Don
September, 2016."

PART 1:

EARLY YEARS

Chapter 1

Pre-School

610 NW 22nd St., Oklahoma City

Until after WWII we lived in the green shingle home of my maternal grandmother, Lena Taylor. Two bedrooms, one bathroom, and a sleeping porch.

In 1944, when I was three-and-a-half, Mom left me in an orphanage in Oklahoma City so she could spend a week with Dad in California before he left for World War II in the Pacific.

My first view of the orphanage was a deserted hall filled with empty bunk beds in formation. Echoes of shouting children outside filtered through half-open windows. A towering nun swathed in black waited and looked down. "Welcome to Saint Anthony's" (not the real name). She didn't smile.

My loving, predictable world was replaced by bunk beds, bullies, and nuns in full habit on patrol.

What weapon did the habit conceal?

I found out. In the play yard, a nun caught me peeing behind a tree and out came a wooden paddle. Another time, another nun, the weapon was the knot at the end of the cord that bound her habit.

The orphanage memory exploded 40 years later. I was on the faculty of the University of Miami medical school and invited to speak at the medical school in Guadalajara, Mexico. On a free morning, my host took me to see Hospicio Cabañas, a UNESCO World Heritage Site, where murals by José Clemente Orozco, one of Mexico's great muralists, decorate the chapel. After I spent an hour admiring, studying, and photographing the murals, our Carmelite Sister guide asked, "Would you like to see our charity work in another section of the Hospicio?"

"*Por supuesto, gracias,*" I answered, and she led us across an interior courtyard to a massive walnut double door. When she opened the door, I was struck speechless by a bolt from the depths of my subconscious that instantly transported me to the orphanage where my mother had left me in August 1944. Thirty bunk beds and a bunch of boys running around. I had repressed that scene for 40 years.

***

I did not realize until I was writing this memoir that my experience at the orphanage was the unlikely first chapter in a life-long love story. Dad had been ordered to leave with his unit from Tinker Field near Oklahoma City for California. From there they would be shipped to an unknown destination in the Pacific. Top Secret: point of departure unknown, destination unknown. Mom bid him goodbye at the train, then returned home and began to network. She called wives whose husbands had already departed for the unknown California destination, located a few who had found their Top-Secret husbands, and learned the location of my dad's outfit after a week of long-distance investigation. He was at a base in Riverside, California, bivouacked with his unit, awaiting departure. Final score: Mom 1, Top Secret 0.

She boarded a train packed with military personnel to search for her husband in Riverside. Standing room only, so she stood. Halfway across Oklahoma, a kind soldier let her sit on the wooden bench for the rest of the three-day trip.

In Riverside she located his unit. They met and arranged to stay in a nearby motel for a week. Their cabin was called Winken, Blinken, and Nod. Near that cabin was the fountain where the happy young couple is sitting in the photograph. When she returned to my grandmother's house, she told me about staying in Winken, Blinken, and Nod. She said later that I asked, "Do they have fairy tales in war?"

"I hope so," she had replied.

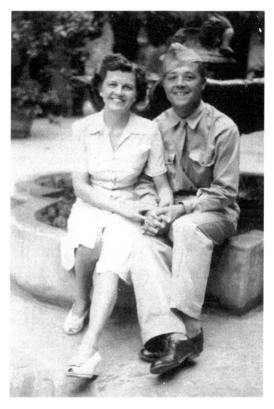

Fig. 1. My mother Rosemary and father Howard, August 1944, in Riverside, California, before my father's embarkation for Saipan.

I had many memorable moments with Mom while Dad was on Saipan—watching thunderstorms from our front porch, learning to fold socks with the "army smile," accompanying her on her job surveying farmers' use of galvanized metal. I still enjoy sitting on the front porch to watch thunderstorms and feel the calm I felt with her.

Daily excitement peaked when the postman arrived with a letter from Dad, although military censors had usually deleted words, lines, or entire paragraphs with scissors. As a joke, Mom and I would occasionally write him a letter and cut out a few lines. She wrote him an anniversary card that featured a picture of the postman in uniform standing beside her, Janet, and me. *A mysterious man in uniform has been visiting Rosemary while her husband is away at war!*

Mom and I slept on the sleeping porch most of the year. A breeze all year, warm quilted blankets in winter. An Oklahoma sleeping porch was the best place to spend the night, except during August. Summers were hot and dry. With no air conditioning, we slept on the driveway when the sleeping porch was too hot. My grandmother Lena stored her rollaway beds in her detached garage. Each night we wheeled our beds onto the driveway and went to sleep. Neighbors did the same on adjacent driveways, and each morning Mom and I awakened to greet the Dodsons as we all stored our beds.

Dad returned from Saipan at the end of 1945. Mom and I drove to Camp Chaffee, Arkansas to greet him when he was discharged. We sat with other families on folding chairs around the edge of a large waiting room. After receiving his discharge papers, each soldier would enter the waiting room a civilian.

Either my facial recognition skills were poor, or I was overexcited. I ran to the wrong man, jumped into his arms, and exclaimed "Daddy!" I was so embarrassed that when the real Dad finally came through the door, I'm sure I didn't give him the welcome he deserved, or I felt.

A few months later, I went with Dad and his friend, Ben Rucker, to see a celebration of the end of WWII at Taft Stadium. Soldiers, sailors, marines, airmen, and military bands marched around the track, accompanied by tanks, jeeps, and howitzers. Fireworks ended the show. The best part was having Dad at my side.

Of course, Dad returned to Janet's world, too. She was now almost two years old. Diapers were made of cloth, provided and cleaned weekly by a diaper service. One afternoon the diaper man arrived to collect Janet's dirty diapers from my grandmother's only bathroom. She led him to the bathroom. The door was locked.

She knocked. "Howard ... Howard ... it's the diaper man."

"Okay, Lena. I'm in the middle of a wipe. I'll open the door in a minute."

Cheeks reddening, my grandmother waited patiently with the diaper man outside the door until Dad emerged.

We then moved to a tiny house not far from my grandmother's house Dad had bought as an investment before the war. The head of my bed abutted the front window. I awoke one morning to spy a large brown tarantula tiptoeing across the front yard. I ran from my bed and asked Mom to capture the hairy creature for me to take to kindergarten. She used a Mason jar for the job.

I suspect that her collaboration then was a harbinger of her support for my future obsession with dissecting euthanized cats and pig embryos at our home during my high school years.

Chapter 2

Elementary Schools

At the age of 4, the first sentence I wrote on Miss Romine's kindergarten blackboard was, "I hate hominy". On a happier note, Miss Romine told Mom that I was the only boy who had ever topped the class in reading.

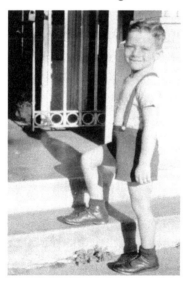

Fig. 2. Age four, first day of kindergarten at Woodrow Wilson Elementary School, Oklahoma City.

Edgar Taylor, Mother's father, was committed to the Central State Hospital in Norman, Oklahoma in 1939, two years after he had suffered a severe stroke. I knew him only during Mom's monthly visits to the hospital, which ended when we moved to Fredericksburg in 1946. He was released from the hospital in the 1950s and committed suicide a short time later.

Mother's brother, Edward Taylor, delivered donuts from a bakery to stores in Oklahoma City, starting at 4:30 a.m. He let me ride in the truck as assistant a couple of times. He also raised rabbits in backyard hutches. He killed himself in about 1960.

Fredericksburg/San Antonio: From Age 5 to 7

Dad was transferred from Oklahoma City to San Antonio as a traveling salesman for Paramount Pictures. After WWII, housing was in short supply throughout the United States. No houses were available in San Antonio, so my parents rented one in Fredericksburg, 70 miles north. Fredericksburg was a quaint German-heritage rural village, an ideal place to enter first grade. Shoes for school were optional, so I often walked to school barefoot.

Neighbors butchered their sheep in a nearby creek bed. Even though they buried the remains, the smell of decay lingered for a couple of weeks.

We lived across the road from the fairgrounds and watched weekend horse races from our front porch.

As in many immigrant German communities, toddlers in cafe highchairs had a small glass of beer on the tray. Since my mother's family on her mother's side was German (Muenchmeyer), I tried to introduce this custom to our family dinners. Mom said, "Nein," with a smile.

In a Main Street record store, I discovered my first country and western music idol, Gene Autry. Listen to "Back in the Saddle Again" sometime.

Fredericksburg in later years became an upscale Texas Hill Country getaway and haven for those who work from home.

The company transferred Dad frequently during these years, so "house hunting" became a weekend family activity. Janet and I rode in the back seat and listened to radio adventure broadcasts. Our favorites were *The Shadow*, ending each week with a creaking door and the deep-voiced narrator warning, "The Shadow knows"; *Sky King* with his airplane *Songbird*; *The Green Hornet*; *The Lone Ranger*; and *Sergeant Preston of the North-West Mounted Police*.

I guess Mom and Dad ran rapidly through each house they inspected to keep Janet and me from exhausting the car battery listening to the radio.

We moved to San Antonio after a few months, but my memories of Fredericksburg have endured longer than those of the "big city." I'm grateful for the post-war housing shortage.

Neighbors across the street in San Antonio were "carnies" and worked in a traveling carnival.

Our Belgian babysitter had a torn photograph she showed Janet and me. Belgium was conquered by the Nazis in 1940 and occupied until late 1944. The babysitter had a black and white photograph, her only memento from her teenage years in Brussels. Unfortunately, a Nazi soldier had posed at her side. She had torn the photograph in half vertically to eliminate him.

Our dentist's office downtown was on the sixth floor of the Medical Arts building, directly across the street from The Alamo. The most hallowed adobe building in Texas history had a galvanized silver steel roof! Even more memorable was that the dentist did not use local anesthesia to drill and fill. I had dentist PTSD for years.

We no longer had to sleep on the driveway to stay cool during hot summer nights. A box fan mounted in an open window had an attached garden hose that dripped water down a screen as the fan blew a moist breeze into the bedroom—an Evaporative Air Cooler that worked well in low Texas humidity. Modern technology!

Dallas/711 Reverchon Drive: From Age 8 to 11

When I was eight, we moved to Dallas. I remember at age nine, while walking home from school with friends, I discovered a naked couple *in flagrante delicto* in the back seat of a parked car on a dirt road. Looking through the back door window I could see the girl's arm wrapped around the guy on top of her. She had a distinctive gold bracelet on her wrist. I hurried home to share the details, as best I knew them, with neighborhood friends. None understood. A week later riding home from school, I recognized the same gold bracelet on the wrist of a girl on our Rosemont *Elementary school* bus. Elementary school? She couldn't have been more than 11 or 12 years old. Seventy years later, I realize that I had probably witnessed statutory rape. At this late date, I can only hope that her life turned out well.

Our family version of "the talk" occurred three years later, when I was 12. My father had been appointed for the task, because Mother never talked with me about sex. Dad's talk was one of extreme mutual discomfort. I remember one sentence he must have gleaned from a 1950s parenting book. "Don, some day you may wake up and find your seed spilled on the bedsheet." By this time, I had already incorporated gentle massage into my bedtime routine, along with brushing my teeth. I knew what he was talking about, but the phrase was pretty weird.

A week later I awoke to find on my bed sheet a furry, firm, brown, lozenge-shaped object about the size of the tip of your little finger. I suspect it was a seed pod Dad had found while he was gardening and hidden beneath my top sheet to stimulate me to initiate the next chapter of "the talk." I didn't, so my sex education was over.

***

I am writing these memories in 2020, during the Covid-19 pandemic. In Dallas I lived through a previous deadly epidemic, infantile paralysis (polio), also caused by a virus that had no vaccine or treatment—the poliovirus. A national poll showed that polio was second only to the atomic bomb as America's greatest fear. Every summer the number of cases soared, leaving thousands of children paralyzed and many dead. The ventilator that assisted breathing during paralysis was the iron lung. In summer my parents prohibited me from swimming in a nearby creek to avoid infection by this mysterious, incurable disease. Normally, when parents forbid something, it becomes more attractive. Somehow, the creek did not. I guess my 10-year-old mind must have balanced a refreshing dip in the creek versus life in an iron lung. A polio vaccine became available in 1955.

4317 Edmondson Avenue, Highland Park

Mom and Dad introduced me to musical theater in 1950— *Brigadoon* and *South Pacific* at Dallas Summer Musical Amphitheater. I owe my lifelong appreciation of live musical performances of all varieties to their gift.

Before we owned a TV set, our family would walk to a closed appliance store in Highland Park Village to watch programs through the window. There I saw General Douglas McArthur give his "Old Soldiers Never Die" speech to a joint session of Congress after he was fired by President Truman in 1951. Boxing, football, and baseball in the front yard were favorite Edmondson activities with Dad.

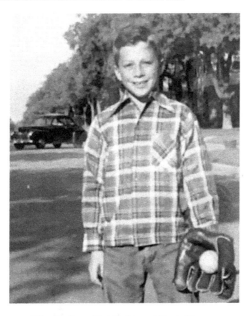

Fig. 3. Age 11, Highland Park, Texas.

During my year at Bradfield Elementary School, my athletic career peaked. I played halfback for the Bradfield Bazookas football team.

Chapter 3

Family Road Trips

After WWII, Americans began to take summer road trips as family vacations. Dad, a traveling salesman, planned ours. When we lived in Dallas, we drove to Cloudcroft, New Mexico and rented a small cabin. Large chain motels and resorts did not appear until the late 1950s. I rode horseback each day and hiked in the hills around our cabin.

A few days later we drove to Carlsbad Caverns, which we first visited at sunset to see the nightly exit of thousands of bats from the cave to feed on airborne insects at night. The bats slept in the cavern during daytime. Carlsbad was discovered at sunset by a lone teenage cowboy, who followed a plume of smoke rising out of the ground, which turned out to be bats flying from the cave.

After we moved to Memphis, our first vacation was a drive through middle Tennessee, to the Hermitage, Rock City, and Ruby Falls.

By then Janet was old enough that she and I played games to entertain ourselves during the ride. We counted bridges and culverts, kept track of out-of-state license plates, and different kinds of farm animals. Other frequent features seen along the highway were barns with a large white "See Rock City" signs painted on the roof—an early marketing venture by the owners of the attraction. We counted those, too.

On a trip to the Smoky Mountains, my best memory was not scenery or culverts, but bears. Families of black bears pawed through garbage barrels along the roadside, surrounded by parked cars and tourist families who stopped to watch and photograph the bears. The danger of bears and people crowded together on highways in national parks was not recognized until many years later. Black bears love watermelon.

One year we drove to Washington, DC. There we toured the National Air Museum (now the Air and Space Museum) and my favorite, the FBI headquarters. At the shooting range in the basement of the FBI building we watched target practice by FBI agents. One of them fired a Thompson submachine gun and nearly cut the target in half.

I asked the agent for the target, but he had already promised it to another boy. About two months later in Memphis, an envelope addressed to me arrived from "Agent Leo B. App." It contained a human full-size target riddled with .45-caliber bullet holes across the middle.

On a trip to New York City, we stayed in a hotel "sample room," a room rented at a lower rate to salesmen to display their products. Though walls were scuffed and scratched, the room was clean. Our shared bath was at the end of the hall. But we were in New York City!

Across the street was an automat, where Dad took us for lunch. This was the predecessor of fast-food restaurants like McDonald's. Food items were displayed in individual small cabinets with glass doors. We would each select a sandwich, piece of pie, or muffin. Dad would insert the change required, and *Voilà!* Here was our meal.

His favorite destination was the Rockettes show in Radio City Music Hall. All of us enjoyed the precision of the choreography and the precision of the Caucasian dancers. Especially Dad.

Chapter 4

Junior High

Memphis: 1625 Tutwiler. From Age 12 to 14

Snowden Junior High

For the Snowden Greenies junior high football team, I was a blocking dummy during team practice. My career high point came when I was sent onto the playing field by Coach Keith for the last play of the season's last game—wearing a numberless practice jersey. Coach Keith made a big impression on the student body at auditorium assemblies, because he always walked onto the stage scratching his crotch.

I was the most unathletic of grandfathers. Non-athlete status lasted a lifetime. I never cliqued. At my 60th high school reunion, an ex-jock ridiculed me when I linked awkwardly to a YouTube presentation while I was serving as MC for the class luncheon. I got him back, though. The YouTube presentation was submitted by an internationally famous poet from our class, Richard Tillinghast, whom I had invited. Richard's fine video performance left the final score Nerds 2, Jocks 1.

Richard's entry in Wikipedia is longer (98 lines) than any other member of our Memphis Central High School class of 1958. Longer even than that of Avron Fogelman (42 lines), businessman, philanthropist, former part-owner of the world series champion Kansas City Royals baseball team, and namesake for the southeast leg of I-240 in Memphis, the Avron B. Fogelman Expressway.

Several times during sixth grade, I invited my classmate and neighbor, Andrea Baker, to see my stamp collection at our home. At a reunion 40 years later, she told me that she had accepted the invitations because she thought my father was cute. Fortunately, he was still alive, and I shared the compliment with him.

Mom and Dad returned from the doctor one afternoon to announce that Janet and I were to be blessed with a sibling. Ultrasound for pregnancy didn't arrive until 1956, so Robert's sex was a mystery.

My favorite solitary pastime was playing with toy soldiers. I was outside building dirt forts one Saturday when the obstetrician called and asked for my father. I told him that he was at the paint store, so he left a message. I had a baby brother.

Plinking in Wolf River bottoms with Buddy Onn and Bob Forrest was my favorite junior high weekend social activity. The garbage dump was located just across Wolf River, so we climbed the abandoned bridge to shoot rats. One Saturday afternoon Buddy shot himself through the right calf practicing his quick draw technic with a cocked .22 LR revolver. We took him to the local GP, who probed the wound, dressed it, and sent him home. No police report, no investigation.

While we lived on Tutwiler, my parents gave me my first dog, an adorable furry, light brown, mixed chow puppy we named "Skippy." After I had learned to take care of him for a few months, Skippy ran out the front door and across Tutwiler, a busy secondary street. I ran after him, calling, "Skippy … Here, Skippy." He ran toward me from the other side of the street and was crushed beneath the tires of a car unable to stop in time. The driver helped me carry dead Skippy to our yard, and that evening Dad helped me bury him. Watching him answer my call and get killed left a painful memory for a long time. I never owned another dog. I did, however, buy an adorable German Shepherd, "Shadow," for my son Keith's eight birthday.

The whole family enjoyed Friday night screenings at the Paramount offices. Dad was branch manager, so he let me celebrate birthday parties with my friends watching movies at the screening room. In subsequent high school class reunions, the private Paramount screenings were my classmates' best memory of me.

Being a film business family made movies a lifelong pastime for all of us. Until the pandemic shutdown in 2020, the Cosford Cinema at the University of Miami was a favorite weekend destination for Magda and me, and we looked forward to its reopening. Times had changed, though—the opening feature in late 2022 was *Bros*.

Chapter 5

High School

Memphis: 1819 Forrest. Ave.

Central High: Grades 10 to 12

I did two stupid things to shake the nerd image. I smoked cigarettes and drank wine. On the positive side, I played Friday night poker at the Chisca Hotel, thanks to Bill Woodmansee, whose father was manager. Woody once snuck us in the back door of the Chisca Club to see Elvis Presley perform, before Ed Sullivan catapulted him to fame. His natural hair color then was light auburn.

During our poker sessions, Woody's father had his catering staff prepare a selection of snacks laid out on a long table—chips, ham and cheese, turkey sandwiches, desserts. When it was my turn to host the group at our home, Mom asked if I wanted her to prepare some snacks. "Sure," I replied. "Just some chips, nuts, and soft drinks. Maybe ham, cheese, turkey sandwiches. And dessert."

I quit smoking the first day I sliced into a smoker's lung with an autopsy knife my second year of medical school. The lung tissue was black as coal, rather than the glistening color of freshly cut ruby red grapefruit. My seven years of teenage smoking could still kill me.

Buddy, Bob Forrest, and I would occasionally buy a bottle of Mogen David wine. We drove north on Thomas Street through a not-quite-ghetto and parked at the curb near a liquor store. Before long a random old man with worn work clothes shuffled along the sidewalk. One of us got out of the car: "Hey Mister! How'd you like to make five bucks?"

"How's that, Mister?"

"Go into the liquor store. Buy a bottle of Mogen David wine. It costs about four dollars. Keep the change."

"Okay, Mister."

Five minutes after giving him a ten-dollar bill, he returned to complete the transaction.

Thomas Street turns into US Highway 51 North. After a 20-minute drive we reached the Ellis Drive-in Theater in Millington. There, in the comfort of my 1950 Plymouth, with its as-advertised "chair-high seats," we watched *Blackboard Jungle* and shared our bottle of Mogen David.

By coincidence, 11 years later my parents bought the Ellis Drive-In after Dad had left Paramount. They converted it to the 51 Twin Drive-In and spent 20 years managing the business. Mom worked in the ticket booth, Dad in the concession stand. Mom's job also included bookkeeping, tax returns, and audits. The interviews I recorded with her include her bravura performance at an in-house IRS audit in Millington. She was a gifted actor.

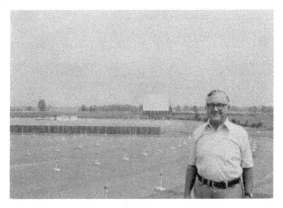

Fig. 4. Millington, 1969.
The proud owner of the
51 Twin Drive-In Theater.

My career vision started to focus at age 14. I wanted to become a general practitioner in a small Arkansas town, like Bald Knob. My role model was Mallory Harwell, a general surgeon in Memphis and Osceola, Arkansas, who flew me to Osceola in his Ryan Navion to watch him operate. On the way back we made an intermediate rest stop, landing on a manicured pasture behind a mansion north of Memphis. I waited in the plane for an hour. Mallory returned to take off for the remainder of our return flight. It took several years and a comment from Mom about her conversations with Mallory's wife for me to understand what the rest stop was.

In 1957 I won second place in the Tennessee state high school state science fair, rewarding my teenage obsession—dissecting euthanized cats and pig embryos in the dilapidated, deserted servants' quarters attached to our garage.

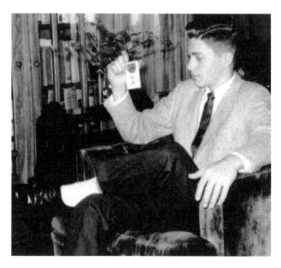

Fig. 5. 1957. Second place, Tennessee state high school science fair.

Although household workers had, for previous owners, lived in the servants' quarters, the space was abandoned when I built my anatomy lab. Folding tables, jars of formaldehyde, no bathroom. It was heaven.

I inaugurated my lab in early 1956. Mom was the accomplice in my dead-animal dissecting career. First, she retrieved dead cats that had been euthanized at the humane shelter. Every Friday afternoon, she drove to the Memphis Humane Shelter with an empty brown cardboard box on the floor of her back seat. After a few minutes, an attendant would return with the box, now containing a dead cat. After she drove home, I would take the box to my laboratory.

When I decided to study fetal (before birth) blood circulation, pigs seemed the ideal subject for investigation. Every few weeks Mom would then drive to the slaughterhouse and wait for a pregnant sow to be slaughtered. Unborn fetal pigs were delivered in a cardboard box to the back floor of her car.

Can you imagine asking your mother to bring dead cats and dead pig embryos to the family home? She did it to support my career dream. The same reason that Caitlan Clark's father enlarged their driveway basketball court into the back yard, so she could practice shooting from well behind the three-point line.

Mom was the goldest standard ever of parental support.

***

Bill Keesling, Buddy, and I spent a few days in November 1956 at a deserted-in-winter Arkansas summer camp, where I had been a counselor. We spent our time hiking through the forest and shooting. Mostly shooting.

On the return Sunday trip to Memphis, at a sharp, unmarked left turn, I rolled my 1950 Plymouth onto its roof in a cotton field outside Newport. The sheriff took us and our pistols (.22 LR, .38 special, and .45 automatic), rifles, and shotguns to the Jackson County Jail. We told our cellmates our story and asked why we might have been locked up.

"You said you boys has some guns? Waiill, somebody robbed a gun store in town. What guns you got?"

I told him and asked, "What kind did they steal?"

".22, .38, and .45 pistols, couple a' shotguns, couple a' rifles."

By the time Dad arrived from Memphis, authorities had established that ours were not the stolen arms.

A Navy cellmate gave us parting advice: "Boys, if ya'll ever steal batt'ries, don't spill th' acid".

He pointed to his navy-blue trousers, pocked by quarter-size holes with underlying blistered red skin.

After the visiting Assembly of God choir invited us to be saved, we were released. When the car was repaired, Dad had it painted turquoise green. From then on, it was "The Easter Egg."

***

During high school, I had typical bouts of adolescent depression. I remember none of the issues, but I do remember the insomnia. I would toss and turn, unable to fall asleep, or awaken in the middle of the night. I went to my parents' bedroom to tell Mom that I couldn't sleep. Dad was always sound asleep, snoring. Mom would put on her robe and walk with me to the front porch, sit on the steps, listen, and talk. About what, I don't remember, but our chats never failed to relieve my anxiety, and I always went back to sleep. Fortunately, my insomnia interrupted their coupling only once—I think.

Dad built a basketball backboard and goal attached to the garage, where he tried to teach me to play. His Oklahoma City Classen High School basketball team had won second place at the national finals in New York City under Coach Hank Iba. Dad was 5'7" tall.

Weekends Dad and I would play golf and tennis. I never developed any of the sports skills he tried to teach. Too bad he wasn't still alive when I learned as an old man to run long distances, including marathons.

My favorite Central High teacher and mentor was Dorothy Green, chemistry. I did take time to thank her during a summer vacation from Stanford. At her modest apartment on Poplar, we sat on her print sofa, and I told her how much she meant to me. Now that I have been a teacher, I know how infrequently that happens, and how much it means.

My girlfriend was Beverly Scott, a gifted soprano. My best friends (after Beverly) were Buddy and Bob Matlock, known as "Bobby Joe," until he finished dental school years later and became "Bob."

Chapter 6

Jobs

Entrepreneur, Lawyer, or Doctor?

Ages 12 and 13

I tramped around the neighborhood as delivery boy for the Memphis *Press-Scimitar* afternoon newspaper. Newsprint rubbed onto my skin, turning hands black by the time I'd finished folding and throwing papers. Mom had Lava hand soap, used by auto mechanics, ready for me at home.

For the duration of a family vacation, I hired as my substitute a 15-year-old next-door neighbor, "Y." Third day on the job, Y stole a car and tried to escape on foot by running up the steps of an elderly customer's house. "Collect for the *Press-Scimitar*," he shouted. She opened the door and he barged past her to run straight for the back door, which is where the police were waiting. On subsequent family vacations I stayed home to cultivate my own paper route.

Ages 13 and 14

I was summer camp counselor at Camp Tahkodah, an Arkansas boys camp. Riflery, boating, tennis, and horseback were my areas of expertise. I had a scar at the center of my back after removal of a mole a few years before. In my introduction to rifle safety, I showed campers the scar and warned them not to point rifles down range while I was replacing targets.

Adrenaline surged in my boating class the time I used the paddle to whack a five-foot-long cottonmouth swimming alongside the boat. The snake went down after the whack, then up. The boat went up after the whack, then down. Snake and boat had both responded to Newton's Laws of Motion, and we were now at eye level. A couple of gentler whacks on the head killed the snake and ended the physics lesson.

Ages 14 to 17

I was grocery bag boy, then checkout clerk, at Food Fair. A grizzled 50-year-old white man gave me a lesson in Southern etiquette at my cash register: I should not have called the Black customer in front of him "Sir."

"No 'ma'am' for Black women, neither."

Ages 18 to 20

During college summers I worked consecutive shifts every day (1) at Memphis Downtown Airport as ground crew (directing small planes after landing and before takeoff) and communications, and (2) at Waterways Marine as deckhand, then night grocery manager.

I was promoted to night grocery manager when the previous manager "N" left to serve a 60-day jail sentence. The minimum wage was $1.00 per hour. I worked 40 hours at each job, earning $80 total—megabucks at the time.

Our lives all include episodes when we remain silent instead of responding to criticism. We realize only later what we should have said. My most memorable example occurred while I was working on the river. Charlie Smith, a gruff, short, round, bald, alleged ex-army major was owner of the company, Waterways Marine. One afternoon he called all hands on deck to read us the riot act. During the performance he singled me out.

"The new night grocery manager [me] left the produce locker in a mess!" he growled. "When N came back"—from his jail sentence—"it was spick and span on my morning inspection today."

To my everlasting regret, I did not reply that while N was cleaning the produce box so well, he and the supply boat operator had failed to load labeled, ready-to-go crates of meat onto the supply boat with other groceries for the large towboat *T. M. Norsworthy*. A capital offence.

I had made the right decision to become a doctor, rather than a lawyer.

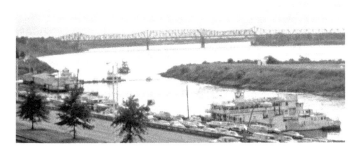

Fig. 6. 1958. Mouth of the Wolf river. Waterways Marine is based on the barge to the left with a small towboat and fuel barge docking perpendicular to Wolf River. The south end of the Memphis Downtown Airport runway is on Mud Island, between the Mississippi and Wolf rivers.

Chapter 7

College

Stanford: 1958 to 1962

I applied only to Stanford because Dad had visited the campus during his one semester at Cal Berkeley before the Great Depression. I recall him remarking, "The campus was heaven. Memorial Church was the most beautiful place I had ever seen."

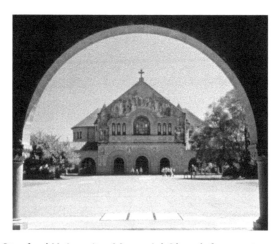

Fig. 7. Stanford University. Memorial Church from entrance arch to the Quad.

In September 1958, I was dropped onto a different planet. Alone on a second-floor motel balcony on El Camino Real, I watched my parents' 1953 Buick join southbound traffic on US 101 to begin the return trip to Memphis. Soon it was time to cross El Camino and meet the other recent arrivals on this new planet.

Public education in the segregated South apparently qualified me for admission to Stanford, perhaps to boost student diversity. Racial desegregation did not reach Stanford until after I had graduated, so faces in the 1962 Stanford Quad yearbook were eerily similar to those from my 1958 Memphis Central High yearbook.

Cultural adaptation was not a one-way street. I contributed to my classmates' worldview by introducing them to country music. Ken DeBevoise couldn't get "Wolverton Mountain" by Claude King out of his head. It inspired him to become a professor at University of Oregon.

My car radio and I drove Sandy Fitch to 8 a.m. chemistry lectures our sophomore year, and he was hooked for a lifetime. He became the Silicon Valley venture capital cognoscente of country music.

Toxic Residue

I struggled for over 50 years to overcome the toxic residue of having been raised in the South.

At age 14, with the first earnings from my paper route, I bought Douglas Southall Freeman's *Lee's Lieutenants*. It was my introduction to Lost Cause Mythology. From that time, I became a serious student of the Civil War, trying to understand the dissonance between books like Freeman's and what I felt.

The toxic residue started with the name of the street where I lived—Forrest Avenue in Memphis. It was named for Nathan Bedford Forrest, a prominent Memphis businessman before the Civil War. His business? Slave trade and real estate. His slave sales lot was located on Adams Avenue downtown, close to the railroad station and river landing.

Since slaves were property, like houses and horses, they could be mortgaged. Combining slave trade and realty was a good business plan. During the Civil War, Forrest rose through the ranks from private to lieutenant general and became one of the best cavalry commanders in the Confederacy. His victories included capture of Fort Pillow, a Union garrison of six hundred soldiers, half Black, on the Mississippi River north of Memphis. About three hundred mostly Black Union soldiers were shot and killed after they surrendered, the infamous Fort Pillow Massacre. After the war Forrest was an early member and Grand Wizard of the first Ku Klux Klan.

So much for my residential street name. I graduated from Memphis Central High School in 1958. As in most southern cities, public schools were still segregated long after the Brown v. Board of Education decision in 1954. There were as yet no laws to enforce the Supreme Court decision, which thus hung like a limp flag for over a decade. One of my teachers emphasized that slavery was not a cause of the Civil War, merely something that distinguished southern cotton production from northern industrial production, like steel in Pittsburgh.

At Stanford my freshman year I was baptized with the nickname "Reb," as in Johnny Reb, the quintessential Confederate foot soldier. The name stuck for years. I had been discharged from the southern segregated educational pipeline as a confused but confirmed subconscious white supremacist.

Racial toxicity boiled over in Memphis after I left. In 1967, two sanitation workers were ground to death in a defective garbage truck. Early attempts to unionize or negotiate salaries and working conditions by Memphis municipal workers were blocked by the mayor, a staunch segregationist and vocal white supremacist. In early 1968, Dr. Martin Luther King, Jr., arrived in Memphis to support Rev. James Lawson and other organizers of the "I Am a Man" strike.

On April 4, King was assassinated.

On April 5, Mike Royko wrote on target in the *Chicago Daily News*: "FBI agents are looking for the man who pulled the trigger and surely they will find him. But it doesn't matter if they do or they don't. They can't catch everybody, and Martin Luther King was executed by a firing squad that numbered in the millions."

Enforcement of Memphis school desegregation began in the early 1970s. City fathers complied by replacing segregated public schools with poorly funded, poorly staffed public schools intended for blacks and those whites who couldn't afford the newly formed private white segregation academies like Briarcrest Christian School, where the Tuouhys sent Michael Oher in *The Blind Side. A Black future NFL star in a school designed to preserve white supremacy?* That's pure Memphis.

In 2009 James Mc Pherson, Pulitzer Prize winning Princeton professor of history, told us in Gettysburg: "My first death threats came in response to my publication of an academic study of southern state school boards at the beginning of the 20th century. The state boards selected only history books that would spread the Myth of the Lost Cause to all public schools."

That answered the question, "Who won the war?" Whoever rewrote and approved the history books. Jim McPherson gave me my Emancipation Proclamation at age 68 in Gettysburg.

I finally recognized what had caused my toxic educational environment.

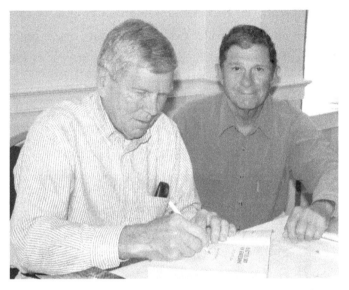

Fig. 8. Gettysburg, 2009. With James M. McPherson, Professor of History at Princeton and Pulitzer Prize-winning author, signing *Battle Cry of Freedom*.

A World of Experience and Possibilities

My major at Stanford was biology, minor German. I studied every night in empty Quad classrooms. Years later, I realized that my time would have been better-spent networking. My occasional after-study rewards were beer, unshelled peanuts, and a hard-boiled egg at the Oasis. In 2018 after SCOTUS declared that discarded peanut shells on the floor were a fire hazard, the "O" closed.

During my freshman year, Mario Prisinzano invited me to Sacramento to spend Thanksgiving with his family. His father, the chief coroner of Sacramento County, arranged for me to watch the on-duty coroner perform autopsies one morning. To camouflage the stench, the doctor lit a strong-smelling cigar before starting work on a decomposed body.

During sophomore year my parents gave me a 1958 VW Beetle, and I drove different routes between Memphis and Stanford two or three times each year.

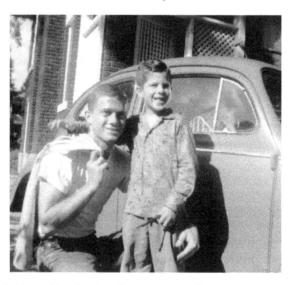

Fig. 9. Memphis, 1961. Robert says goodbye as Don leaves for Stanford in his 1958 VW Beetle.

My best friend, Dick Tully, flew to Memphis to join me for one trip to Stanford after he had finished his Wall Street summer internship. Dick was the most refined person either I or my parents had ever met. Courteous, thoughtful, soft-spoken, well-mannered, prep school diction and pronunciation. He'd never seen the South before, so I drove us through Vicksburg, Natchez, Ferriday, and New Orleans, and then up through interminable Texas. Somewhere near Amarillo, we stopped for Texas chili at a small diner. Our Texas-size waitress could have been a roustabout in a nearby oil field. When we finished the chili, she swaggered to the table: "Waiill boys, haa-ow wuz it?" Dick delicately wiped his lips with his napkin, smiled, and looked up at her. "Very tasty, thank you."

One Christmas two friends rode with me nonstop from Stanford to Memphis. To make room for three of us and our stuff, one had to lie on duffle bags piled on the back seat as we drove. Passing trucks was a challenge in a fully loaded 36 HP VW through the mountains. The car crept to the top of each hill on the two-lane highways. Acceleration finally began at the crest, and that's when the slower acceleration of trucks let me get around them.

In an Arizona sleet storm, wipers couldn't scrape ice from the front windshield, so the passenger leaned outside the sunroof and wiped it by hand as we headed east. Map reading and a sense of direction were essential driving skills before GPS.

Sophomore year I met Allene in German class. Junior year I was elected to Phi Beta Kappa. Senior year I graduated a virgin. With Great Distinction.

The Stanford years brought into perspective a new physical and human world of experience and possibilities. Physician, yes—Bald Knob, no.

In 1962 I married Allene, and we moved to Baltimore.

Chapter 8

Medical School at Johns Hopkins (1962-1966)

I thought I was well armored for medical school, academically and emotionally. After all, I had watched live surgery and dissected cats and fetal pigs since high school and observed autopsies since college.

What blindsided me was how my feelings of sympathy were blunted during some medical training. For example, my cadaver in gross anatomy lab my first year was that of an elderly, emaciated woman who had died from ovarian cancer. The malignancy had seeded the peritoneal surface of her intestines with a white, irregular coating of cancer nodules. Her intestines were encased in friable concrete just beginning to harden. Did I wonder about the life she had lived? Or the agony of her death? No. What concerned me were the extra hours I would have to spend on my futile dissection of intestines encased in cancer and how much her normal intestinal anatomy had been obliterated.

Baltimore 1962 - 63

We lived in a student-house staff complex called The Compound. The surrounding neighborhood was a ghetto, poor, but safe at that time. The Compound is now rubble beneath a parking garage, the neighborhood less safe.

Our furnishings were minimalist. In fact, my third year we entertained my professor-mentor, Dr. Frank B. Walsh, and his wife Josie using an upside-down cardboard packing box as our dining table.

Dr. Walsh, who was 70 when we met, became the closest, dearest friend, role model, teacher, and father-figure that a lowly medical student could ever have. He embodied the best of my Hopkins training experience. Born in Oxbow, Saskatchewan in 1895, he accompanied the Canadian Army to Belgium in World War I. Wounded and gassed at Ypres, he returned to Canada to recuperate and finish medical school. He first entered general practice in remote Saskatchewan and liked to tell me that he had "pulled more teeth than any neuro-ophthalmologist in the world."

His humility glowed even before the most sophisticated neurologists and neurosurgeons: "Doctor, those two eye movements are as different as chalk and cheese," was one of his favorite sayings. Once, when a New York patient insisted on addressing him as "Doc," he turned to me, "I'd rather she call me 'Frank.'"

He founded the subspeciality of neuro-ophthalmology with publication of his classic *Clinical Neuro-Ophthalmology* in 1947. Dr. Walsh wrote the second edition during a period when he had left Wilmer for private practice with Charlie Iliff on Mount Vernon Square. One of the reasons he wrote the new edition then, he explained to me, was to generate income to pay for his first wife's terminal illness, a brain tumor.

One of my duties during electives and summers in the mid-1960s was to assist him with writing and editing the third edition of The Book, now co-authored by William F. Hoyt. I got my first lesson in cut-and-paste, long before the computer era. Dr. Walsh had his editor prepare a complete single-page copy of the second edition. Using scissors and scotch tape, he would cut what he didn't want to keep from each page and replace it with a freshly typed piece from his vintage Underwood typewriter. With Dr. Walsh that year I co-authored a study published in the Archives of Ophthalmology, "Oral Contraceptives and Neuro-Ophthalmological Interest."

He was a living lesson in aging well, the only physician I ever saw take an afternoon nap on the sofa in his office. At age 83 I still follow his lead, snoozing on my bed instead.

Golf at the Elkridge Country Club was his favorite pastime. One hundred and thirty-yard drives straight as an arrow off every tee. Partnered frequently with Howard Naquin, veteran of D-Day and prominent private ophthalmologist, and A. Earl Walker, world-renowned Professor of Neurosurgery at Hopkins, he occasionally invited me to join them as a fourth.

One evening he invited Allene and me to accompany Josie and him to dinner at the Elkridge Club. At the buffet table I dropped a piece of cheese on the floor. As I bent to pick it up, Josie stepped forward. "That's all right," she said. "I'll take care of it," deftly kicking the dropped cheese under the table.

The three-volume third edition of *Clinical Neuro-Ophthalmology* was published in 1969, when Dr. Walsh was 74. He sent me a signed copy and graciously cited my help in the acknowledgments. My main contribution had been researching and rewriting the section on color vision, which he preferred not to touch. Both he and the Wilmer color vision expert approved my work before it was sent to the publisher.

Once while Bill Hoyt was visiting Baltimore to work on The Book, I arranged to take him to the airport for his return flight to San Francisco. Because I had lived on the peninsula for four years at Stanford, I had considered applying for residency at the University of California San Francisco, where he was a professor.

"After Stanford, I've thought about living in the Bay area. Would residency at UCSF give me better connections for practice there?" I asked.

"Since you are interested in academic practice, I would advise residency at a top-notch department elsewhere. If you started at Cal, the faculty would always remember you as the bumbling beginner who made his fair share of mistakes."

I followed his advice.

In 1978 I visited Dr. Walsh for the last time in Baltimore, where he was dying alone of lung cancer. Josie suffered from dementia and had returned to Canada to live in a nursing home. I had been at Bascom Palmer for five years and was becoming an ophthalmology ambassador to Latin America. When I entered his apartment I noted that he was reading David McCullough's new (1977) masterpiece about the Panama Canal, *Path Between the Seas*—the very same book that I was then reading in Miami! He died a few months later at age 83.

At the corner of Monument and Wolfe was the entrance to the Women's Clinic, next to the Pathology Department pick-up bay. One sunny Sunday morning while I walking to Welch Library, I passed an unforgettable scene, which I write about in chapter 24.

Farther east on Monument Street was a Polish/Italian neighborhood, where we walked on weekends to restaurants, Frank Testani's bar, movies, and duck pins. Our best Polish friends, Charlie Schimunek and his wife, owned a funeral home. Their whole clan was full of life.

On October 22, 1962, we watched President Kennedy's Cuban Missile Crisis speech at Roger and Betsy Gstalder's next door. Unlike us, they had a TV.

We drove to Chancellorsville VA, the evening of May 2, 1963, to be at the exact place and time of Stonewall Jackson's fatal wounding exactly a century before. The only other person there was Jesse C. James from El Campo, TX.

Our best contemporary friends were Pat and Carol Wilkinson, who became Darrell's godparents. Pat and I were born 20 miles apart in Oklahoma. We both went to Stanford. We met for the first time in the registration line at the Johns Hopkins medical school. We both selected ophthalmology as our specialty. He finished his residency at Wilmer. I came to Wilmer as chief resident the year after. We both selected retina-vitreous as our sub-specialty.

Coincidence followed us for decades like The Shadow with its creaking door, climaxing at the annual Wilmer alumni meeting. Our independent scientific papers on the program had exactly the same title: "Pseudophakic Retinal Detachment!"

I told the audience: "If either of us develops crushing substernal chest pain radiating to the left elbow, both of us should be admitted to the coronary ICU."

Pat became Chairman of Ophthalmology at the Greater Baltimore Medical Center.

***

Will, Allene, and I took a two-week camping trip to Montreal, the Gaspé Peninsula, New Brunswick, Maine, and Pittsburg. I failed to tighten cloth straps securing the rooftop rack during a New Brunswick rainstorm, and it slid onto the highway, broken. Switching from driver to passenger in the VW bug, I balanced wet sleeping bags and luggage on my lap for the rest of the trip to Pittsburg, where Paramount had transferred my father.

We arrived late at night, so the scene that greeted Mom the next morning from her kitchen window was our trio in three sleeping bags on a tarp in the back yard.

That evening my family gathered in the living room to welcome Allene, Will, and me to their new home. Dad fell asleep in the middle of the floor, snoring loudly, as was his custom.

1964-65

Darrell was born. We had sort of decided to name him after Will, so the birth announcement anticipated his arrival as "William Darrell." We changed the name to "Darrell Howard" before he was born. Allene and I introduced him to camping at Washington Monument State Park, the Maryland Hunt Cup, and sailing on Chesapeake Bay.

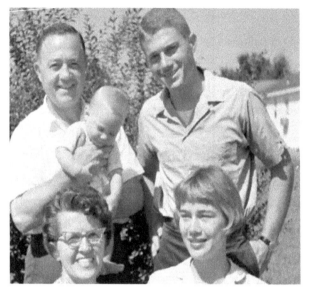

Fig. 10. Millington, 1965. Howard, Darrell, Don, Rosemary, Allene.

Psychiatry and Sailing

Spring quarter senior year was a glorious time for me. Our newborn son Darrell was healthy, internship and residency were confirmed, and my only courses were surgery in the morning and psychiatry in the afternoon. For the first time in years, I felt free to do what I wanted. So I took sailing instead of psychiatry.

I reported to the psychiatry secretary at the Phipps Psychiatric Clinic each afternoon and signed the attendance register. The secretary checked my name and told me where my assigned seminar was located. I don't think she ever sent a copy of the attendance list to the instructors. I left the building, walked to our apartment, wrapped six-week-old Darrell in his blanket, put him in a Clorox box, and drove with him and Allene to a marina on South River near Annapolis. There I rented a 12-foot catboat for $3.00 an hour and taught myself to sail. I can't imagine six weeks of psychiatry therapy doing more for us than our six weeks of psychiatry sailing.

First, Allene received her M.A. degree from Goucher. Second, I gained skills that let me later rent a 41-foot Morgan ketch in the BVI to spend a week with my brother Robert (see chapter 13) and a week in the USVI with Buddy Onn, his wife Shirley, and Darrell. Finally, Darrell acquired a lifelong passion for sailing, which also led to his professional career.

In 1966, I received my M.D. from Johns Hopkins University School of Medicine.

Chapter 9

Internship in Internal Medicine, Vanderbilt University Hospital

Nashville: 153 Haverford Ave. duplex. 1966—1967

Call schedule for most rotations was 36 hours in hospital, 12 hours off, so my year in Nashville was mostly a blur. My best internship lesson: a five-minute shower is more revitalizing than a two-hour nap.

Lara was born that year. As part of the medical family, I was invited to the delivery room by the obstetrician. Fortunately, the doctor asked me to wait outside the door until after the delivery.

I waited … and waited. Still, no newborn cries. Shouts from inside the delivery room: "Take her down. Take her down." Equipment clattered, then silence. Finally came the first loud, healthy cries. The umbilical cord had prolapsed, and Lara was brought into the world under general anesthesia via Dührssen cervical incisions.

My only personal obstetrics experience during this year of internal medicine training came in the driveway to the Vanderbilt Hospital Emergency Department one afternoon. No obstetrics resident was in the ED, so nurses rushed me to an old black Chevrolet, where a screaming mother was giving birth in the back seat. Unfortunately, the baby was stillborn.

In 1966, as the Vietnam War was escalating, I joined the U.S. Navy Medical Corps Reserve and retired in 1977. In 2004, Magda's older son Dax used my Navy career to win a dispute that helped his wife Marion to be issued a green card. An immigration agent wanted assurance that Marion's permanent residency sponsors were solvent, so he asked Dax to bring him my federal tax return. I told Dax that I couldn't risk identity theft by handing my tax return to a stranger. The agent told Dax at his next visit that he had been a United States Marine and would not steal my identity. Dax immediately countered, "My father was a commander in the United States Navy. He won't give you his tax return." Marion's application was approved.

Contributing to a Patient's Death

Ophthalmology doesn't often involve life and death decisions or death of a patient, but internal medicine does. While I was an intern in internal medicine at Vanderbilt, I faced many such situations, which I usually handled well. One I did not.

I was at the end of a 36-hour shift at the VA hospital. At 6 p.m. I could go home, eat, and sleep. My admission patient was a 50-year-old career Army non-com, Willie Gordon (not his real name), who suffered end-stage kidney failure and needed peritoneal dialysis, the final treatment possible in the era before hemodialysis and renal transplant. In peritoneal dialysis, fluid (the dialysate), containing a healthy balance of nutrients and ions, is passed into the peritoneal cavity with a catheter. This cavity is the potential space formed by a continuous membrane lining the internal surface of the abdominal organs, including the stomach. Dialysate, when passed into the peritoneal cavity, removes toxins, adjusts fluid balance, and balances sodium, potassium, phosphorous and other ions with those in the blood stream, just as a normal kidney does.

With Gordon's head elevated in his hospital bed, under aseptic conditions, I inserted the dialysis tube into the catheter that had been placed by the surgery resident two weeks before. The tube was now in his peritoneal cavity, so I let the dialysate drip in. The patient was comfortable, breathing normally, with normal temperature, pulse and blood pressure.

It was 6:15 p.m., and my shift was finished. I greeted the sergeant's wife, who was entering the unit for her usual Sunday evening visit. "Good night, Mrs. Gordon," I said, then headed for my car.

When I returned for my shift the next day, the head nurse told me that Sgt. Gordon died an hour after I had left the hospital. Mrs. Gordon had prepared her husband's favorite low-sodium dish, chicken breasts soaked in buttermilk, then oven-roasted. Gordon smiled and smacked his lips as he downed every bite of the delicious meal. By 7 p.m. the pressure of the dialysate compressed his engorged stomach. He vomited, aspirated the chicken dinner, and suffocated. I had neglected to write an NPO order before I left the hospital. With this order, nurses would have prohibited any food intake.

The Heimlich maneuver, which could have saved Gordon's life, was not described until seven years later.

After internship I worked as a temporary physician in nearby Woodbury. Staff doctors frequently asked me to interpret patient EKGs. I gladly complied but didn't mention that EKG interpretation was taught during residency, not internship.

Forty years after internship I returned to Nashville to run the Country Music Marathon.

Chapter 10

Residency in Ophthalmology

Boston: 146 Palfrey St., Watertown, MA: 1967–1970

Harvard: Mass. Eye and Ear Infirmary (M.E.E.I.)

Johns Hopkins: Wilmer Eye Institute

Sledding down Palfrey Hill was our favorite family winter recreation. We carried the sleds from our house up 50 yards to the crest of the hill and launched our downhill glide, arms around toddlers, Darrell and Lara, whooshing past our house for another 50 yards.

One disadvantage of a small house on a steep street didn't become apparent until spring. We parked our two cars parallel to each other, one on the short driveway, the other just downhill. Our bedroom was above the garage.

We were awakened in the middle of the night by a loud crash outside our window, followed by the sound of grinding, clanking metal and shattering glass. Someone had released a car parked on Palfrey Street uphill and let it roll down in neutral, gathering speed until it broadsided our Plymouth on the driveway, which rolled over, crashing into the side of our VW camper, a perfect billiard combination shot. Fortunately, there was no damage to our downhill neighbor's house. Nevertheless, our entire fleet had been wiped out.

Anti-Vietnam War protests were widespread. I was busy in residency, but Allene, a teacher at Dundalk Elementary, participated frequently. I joined her for at least one, on Boston Common.

At the time of my residency in the late 1960s, there were two attending surgeons on the MEEI faculty who still did not wear surgical gloves, which had been introduced at Johns Hopkins 50 years earlier. One of the most widely acclaimed glaucoma surgeons in the world, Paul Chandler (1896–1987), opined "our fingers would be less sensitive with gloves."

All eye surgery patients were admitted to the hospital for a few days: seven to 10 for retinal detachment repair, and three to five for cataract extraction. By the 1990s all eye surgery patients were operated as outpatients, without admission to the hospital.

My residency partner was Deborah Pavan Langston. Normally each resident surgeon would be assisted by an older attending surgeon from the community or faculty. However, our eye service had just acquired its first operating microscope, an ungainly portable model wheeled into the operating room and adjusted manually to accommodate the surgeon at the head and the assistant at the side. No attending surgeon had ever used the operating microscope, relying instead on special spectacles (loupes) for magnification during surgery. The attending surgeons were reluctant to enter this new surgical world and were glad to observe from outside the sterile field, while Debbie and I assisted each other on all our cases. We thus doubled the usual resident operating experience. Debbie became a star cornea and cataract surgeon and continued her landmark research career at Harvard.[2]

***

Steve Guzak (1938–2021) was my best friend in Boston. We spent many happy evenings together with all our children at their home in Winchester listening to music on Steve's reel-to-reel tape recorder and admiring Karen's abstract oil paintings.

Steve and I worked together on a project to examine the retinal burn to the macula suffered by people who had looked at the sun during a solar eclipse that passed over Boston. We received one referral from the gynecology resident at the Massachusetts General Hospital. The patient was a young woman who had been sunbathing nude on her terrace during the eclipse. She heard later on TV that people might get *rectal*

---

2. https://eye.hms.harvard.edu/deborahpavanlangston

burns from the eclipse, and she wanted to make sure hers was okay.

Steve and I also published a study that irritated many oculoplastic surgeons. "Loss of Vision after Repair of Orbital Floor Fractures" in Archives of Ophthalmology was the first description of a rare, potentially disastrous complication after repair of relatively common blunt trauma (e.g., punch from a fist) around the eye. Postoperative bleeding could lead to increased pressure in the orbit that closes the artery supplying the eye, causing blindness.

Orbital surgeons had to develop new postoperative routines that monitored vision at regular intervals. Since the operated eye was covered by a pressure bandage, this new routine required more postoperative care and time. Because of its infrequency, many surgeons had never encountered the complication, and they considered the new postoperative vision examinations an unnecessary waste of time.

July 29, 1969: With Schramsberg champagne, Allene and I watched the *Apollo 11* moon landing on our own TV.

Ed Maumenee (1913-1998), Chairman of Ophthalmology at Johns Hopkins, called one afternoon while I was working in the MEEI general eye clinic to ask if I would be chief resident at the Wilmer Institute. I accepted and became the only Wilmer chief resident who had not served the first three years of residency in the Wilmer program.

The impression I left on Harvard and the Massachusetts Eye and Ear Infirmary during my three years of residency is best captured on my diploma, which got my name wrong, Don *Harold* Nicholson instead of Don Howard Nicholson. *Así es como es.*

Baltimore: Wilmer Chief Resident 1971–1972

Wilmer residents were trained to be fiercely independent, relying on their own judgement and surgical skill, rather than seeking specific faculty guidance. Halfway through my chief resident year, a teenage high myope with a retinal detachment in her only remaining eye came under my care. I performed the best retinal detachment operation I could and was satisfied with the surgical result and her early postoperative period. In the second week, however, vitreous inflammation and scarring redetached the retina—massive vitreous retraction, it was then called. After examination, I felt that a second operation had a chance of reattaching the retina. I was more inclined to seek faculty help than a three-year foundation of Wilmer culture might have instilled, so I asked Bob Welch (1927-2021), an accomplished faculty retinal surgeon to help me with her surgery.

After a thorough examination of the patient's retina, he turned to me: "No, Don. You can do it." My reoperation did not reattach the retina, and the girl remains blind.

Since I assisted all second- and third-year residents with their operations, I was able to evaluate the skill of each on multiple occasions. I was particularly concerned about the skill and dexterity of one, whom I will name "X." Near the end of his training, I asked him to come to my office for a confidential conversation.

"X," I said, "I really like you and have enjoyed operating with you. However, I'm worried. I've assisted many residents with many operations, and, in my opinion, your surgical skill is well below average. I think it's in your best interest to choose a non-surgical subspecialty, like neuro-ophthalmology."

Instead, X became a nationally recognized corneal and anterior segment surgeon—one of the most demanding, delicate fields of eye surgery.

Returning from a weekend camping trip, we stopped at a car wreck on US-40 outside Frederick, MD. A teenage girl lay unconscious on the median. I maintained her airway with a tongue depressor until the ambulance arrived. Her uninjured anesthesiologist father, the driver, had stood frozen in shock. His daughter survived.

PART 2:

MIDDLE YEARS

Chapter 11

Bascom Palmer Eye Institute

University of Miami School of Medicine 1972-1994

1972: Assistant Professor

We rented 275 W. Mashta Dr., then purchased 769 Allendale Rd., both on Key Biscayne.

When I arrived 10 years after its founding, Bascom Palmer was the youngest, most exciting center of academic ophthalmology in the United States. Within a year, however, I recognized one obvious deficiency. Not a single faculty member or resident spoke Spanish, and there was no program to integrate Spanish into education and patient care, even though the Freedom Flight program from Cuba still operated until 1973. Miami was becoming bilingual. Bascom Palmer was not.

The faculty members at Bascom Palmer were each at the top of their subspecialty field: retina-vitreous, glaucoma, pediatric ophthalmology, cornea, cataract, macula, neuro-ophthalmology. Instead of becoming the bottom rung on a high ladder, I decided to develop a new subspecialty —International Ophthalmology.

How did an ophthalmologist born in Oklahoma and raised in Texas and Tennessee become obsessed with the Spanish language to the point that it became a career focal point? The answer is one specific incident at one specific hour. I had been at Bascom Palmer only a few months and operated in the Jackson Memorial Hospital operating rooms, where the scrub area connected with two operating rooms, one to either side. The swinging door between scrub area and OR was often left open, allowing surgeons scrubbing to overhear a conversation in one OR while they scrubbed for a case in the other. I was scrubbing and overhearing.

In the adjacent OR a retinal detachment repair had just begun under local sedation anesthesia, meaning that the patient was awake and mildly sedated, the eye having been anesthetized by a local anesthetic injected behind the eye. His face was covered by surgical drapes. The surgeon was Professor Victor Curtin (1925–2016), backup for Bascom Palmer Eye Institute founder, Edward Norton, M.D. (1922–1994). The patient was a Cuban in his sixties, who spoke no English. Neither Victor, nor the anesthesiologist, the resident, nor any nurse in the OR that day spoke Spanish. Yes, Virginia, in 1972 Miami operating rooms there were days when none of the surgical team spoke Spanish. The patient apparently moved his head. "Be still, now," said Victor calmly. The patient moved again. "Don't move," a bit louder. At this point someone may have tried a mangled "*No se mueve.*" The patient was still moving, now mumbling in Spanish.

"Don't move your head." Not quite a shout but getting there. Victor was speaking louder and louder to a frightened, uncomfortable patient, face covered, who couldn't understand a word of English. Continuing to scrub, I saw my father on an operating table surrounded by gowned and masked strangers, one of whom was shouting at him in a foreign language. In a dozen lifetimes I could not have found a stronger incentive to study Spanish.

In 1975 Allene and I divorced while she was finishing her J.D. at University of Miami Law School.

I learned that I had a gift for Romance languages. I began planning *El Curso Interamericano de Oftalmología Clínica*, continued studying Spanish, and started learning Portuguese.

I supplemented Berlitz and Inlingua classes with informal tutors—Maria from Buenos Aires and Ana from Fortaleza. They were a big help, although I had to eliminate traces of *lunfardo* from my Spanish.

1977: Associate Professor

During a trip to Santiago, Chile in 1977, I developed an interest in Latin American art for defensive reasons—I didn't want to fill another bag with travel mementos. Instead, by expressing an interest in local artists, my host or spouse was always able to guide me.

In 1979 I founded and began directing *El Curso Interamericano de Oftalmología Clínica*, a course in clinical ophthalmology with simultaneous interpretation (English to Spanish) for practitioners who understand spoken Spanish better than English. By 2019, El Curso attracted over seven hundred registrants annually to Miami from Latin America, the Caribbean, and Spain. A virtual edition in 2021 had seven thousand registrants. How did Spain get into the mix? When Franco was dictator, he eliminated English from all schools throughout Spain, elementary through graduate school. Thus, ophthalmologists of my generation who had not studied abroad could not understand English-language ophthalmology congresses or courses. I added Spain to my mailing list, and within a year, Spanish ophthalmologists comprised 20 percent of our registrants.

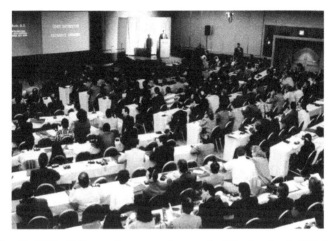

Fig. 11. 1994. *El Curso Interamericano de Oftalmología Clínica.*

The Curso years gave me my best practice at improving my Emotional Quotient (see chapter 23). Socializing with hundreds of friends and colleagues from many countries for a week each year at Curso and at their national congresses at other times drew me out of my "academic success and achievement" addiction and helped me grow close to dozens of new friends.

For the foreseeable future, *El Curso Interamericano de Oftalmología Clínica* will continue to be the educational bridge between U.S. and Latin American ophthalmology. The seedling I planted in 1979 thrives.

Also in 1979, my first book, *Ocular Pathology Update,* was published. I gave my mother a copy on the first Mother's Day after its publication, a small tangible memento of all she had devoted to my career. On my visit to their home in Millington a year later, she told me, "Don, that is a lovely book, I'm so proud of you. I keep it on my bedside table. Whenever I can't go to sleep, I read another few pages, then doze right off." I may ask the publisher to run another printing and promote the book as a nonaddictive soporific. It wouldn't be the first time that I interfered with the publication schedule for this book. In the manuscript I included an acknowledgement to my secretary for her help preparing the book. She divorced during publication, and I had to stop the press to change her last name.

In 1980, Miami burned. Black smoke billowed into the sky from Overtown and Liberty City, centers of the McDuffie riots. I could see massive clouds of smoke from my office May 30, from Darrell's fishing boat on Biscayne Bay May 31, and from the air June 1, as I flew from MIA to a medical meeting.

In 1982, while I was in Cordoba for a conference, Argentina invaded the Falkland Islands and declared war against Great Britain—on April Fools' Day. Cordoba erupted like *Carnaval*—patriotic street celebrations, horns, waving flags. This enthusiastic show of support reminded me of the public exuberance in Miami when the Mariel boatlift began in 1980. Celebrations didn't last long for either.

In 1983 Magda Sara and I married.

Ophthalmologists love ski meetings. Usually with our children, we went to Sun Valley, Aspen, Vail, or Snowmass. Magda was afraid of heights, so her first few outings in Sun Valley were confined to the beginner slope. She had a petite, form-fitting, bright yellow ski suit that shone like a beacon. We called and whistled to her on the Bunny Slope from our lift as it ascended Bald Mountain. David Singer, a good friend and superb skier, convinced her to let him guide her down from the highest peak. Her positive attitude brought dense fog. The morning they went up Old Baldy, fog was so thick Magda couldn't see her ski tips, much less the bottom of the mountain. After her first foggy run, the sky and her acrophobia cleared.

1985: Professor

Magda and Kaki Lopez celebrated my promotion to full professor with a soiree behind our home at 1025 Andora. Pit Bar-B-Q set up their serving line, and everyone came—neighbors, friends, family, colleagues, three-piece band, stripper.

Yes, they hired a stripper for me.

All was mellow until the stripper started climbing on top of me poolside. Pregnant Magda charged, signaling, and shouting: "CUT!! CUT!!" I'm sure that's what she signaled. I'm not sure that is what she shouted. When I saw her charging, I dove into the pool—glasses, clothes, shoes, wallet, the works.

Keith was due to be born a few weeks after the party, unfortunately at a time that conflicted with my invitation to the Dominican Republic to receive the Order of Christopher Columbus.

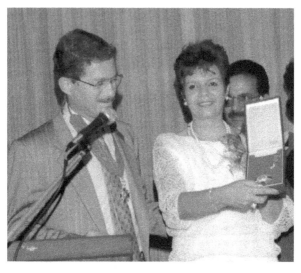

Fig. 12. October 1985. Order of Christopher Columbus, presented by the government of the Dominican Republic.

Magda was understandably upset that I had to abandon her a short time before her due date. I was saved by a medical student from Brazil, Luiz Geraldo Assis, who agreed to stay in our house with Magda and take her to the hospital if she went into labor. In case there wasn't time, Luiz brought with him sterile scissors, clamp, and umbilical tape. Fortunately, Keith waited to appear until I had returned. Rather than Magda's obstetrician, Luiz became Keith Miguel's godfather and a dear friend to all of us.

Medicine has advanced so much since I retired that I'll mention only briefly my practice years. My care for patients with pediatric ocular cancer, for example, seems no different than that a hundred years ago. I practiced during the Neanderthal Era of retinoblastoma treatment.

We had only two treatments for this cancer: removal of the eye (enucleation), or whole-eye irradiation, which itself damages vision. Since I retired, the advances in genetics research and new treatments that save the eye have revolutionized the outcome of retinoblastoma treatment. It is now the pediatric cancer with the highest cure rate in the United States, and useful vision is preserved in the majority of patients. All research leading to this point has been clinical observation of patients and treatments by practicing ophthalmologists, not experiments with animals.

Here are four patients whom I will always remember.

The first was a typical patient, a three-year old boy with retinoblastoma whose eye I enucleated. His parents sent annual photographs and notes. They always eliminated activities that could injure his remaining eye. In high school he became a state champion fencer and won a college scholarship in the sport.

A more unusual patient was a five-year-old boy with a lump under the skin of his right upper lid. My biopsy showed that the tumor was neuroblastoma, a malignant tumor that develops from immature nerve cells. The experts in evaluation and treatment of this cancer were at St. Jude Children's Research Hospital in Memphis. They accepted him with full, free evaluation and treatment for the child and free accommodations for parents and child. My mother in Memphis met the family at the airport and drove them to St. Jude. The initial evaluation was optimistic, but communication from the treatment team then ceased. I hope he made it.

Next is a three-year-old girl whom I thought had vitreoretinal inflammatory disease, perhaps due to toxoplasmosis. After I performed a vitrectomy, histopathology showed retinoblastoma. In consultation with oncologists and other vitreoretinal surgeons, we decided that, perhaps, systemic chemotherapy could destroy the cancer. She received a full course and the tumor disappeared.

We were so optimistic that I wrote a case report, which passed peer review and was accepted for publication by the American Journal of Ophthalmology. The mother took her daughter to Mexico to visit relatives, and she missed two follow-up visits. When she returned after three months, the eye was filled with cancer, and I had to enucleate it. I called to stop the AJO article, which was never published. Many battles, a few victories.

The high point of my career was operating on my father's cataract.

In his early seventies, Dad developed gradual loss of vision in his right eye. He had a traumatic retinal scar in the same eye, so I assumed that the asymmetric progression of the cataract may have been related to trauma (college boxing). We waited until his loss of vision interfered with driving, then proceeded with surgery. The operation was uneventful technically, but most rewarding emotionally, a perfect result. I was able to give something back to the man who had given me so much.

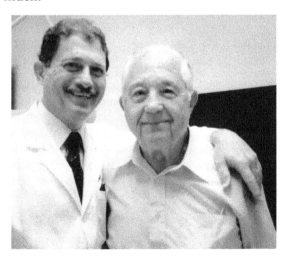

Fig. 13. Dad and his cataract surgeon.

In late 1985 Miguel Diaz, Magda's father, visited Miami from Cuba, sponsored by the Red Cross, for a medical tune-up and to tell his five daughters good-bye.

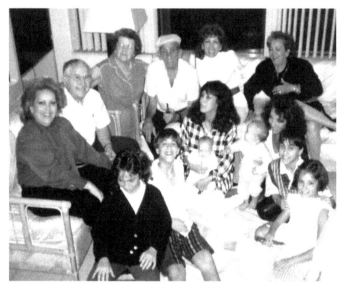

Fig. 14. December 1985. Miguel Diaz visit to Miami with his daughters, their children, and my parents.

From Keith's birth through teenage years, we often attended ophthalmology meetings together. I was invited to speak at 85 conferences and congresses in 19 countries during that time. While I worked, Magda and Keith shopped and played, and we added a few days' vacation before or after most meetings. During his toddler years, we didn't go far. At the Spanish Congress in 1989, Keith was three. We stayed in

Torremolinos, ate tiny clams (*coquinas*) and barnacles (*percebes*), and built sandcastles.

The next year, we wanted to take him to the beach at Matheson Hammock, two miles from our home in Coral Gables. He gathered his traveling gear for the airport because he knew that to get to the beach, one must take an airplane.

By the time Keith was five, we had perfected our exploration strategy. Our favorite base was Seattle. Five meetings over ten years let us explore Wahington, Oregon, Montana, and British Columbia.

We always took our trips to the northwest in August, to avoid the constant Seattle rain. Magda and I took a few of these trips alone, the most memorable to see Seattle Opera's production of Richard Wagner's four operas that comprise *The Ring Cycle*—17 hours spaced over four nights. Each night we both eagerly awaited the next episode. After the last, we were sorry there wasn't another.

Chapter 12

Overseas Adventures, 1972-1994

Gunpoint

I was robbed at gunpoint only once. In 1977, I skipped a group stop in São Paulo to visit Rio de Janeiro by myself. Alone in one of the world's most exotic cities, I began to explore and test the results of Ana's Portuguese instruction.

I was riding the single-car tram to the iconic Cristo Redentor statue. About a third of the way up the mountain, three teenage boys emerged from the trees and stopped the tram. One pointed a .45 automatic pistol at us six passengers. While two accomplices collected watches and wallets from the other passengers, I slipped passport and travelers' checks from my sport coat vest pocket. I was able to rejoin my colleagues in São Paulo the following night. I never saw Cristo Redentor, but I did get to practice my Portuguese by filing a police report.

Smuggler

After the Pan American Congress in Chile in 1977, I decided to visit Argentina. Bill Montalbano (1940–1998), a good friend, had lived in Buenos Aires as Latin American correspondent for the *Miami Herald*, so I asked him for travel tips. He listed his favorite hotel in Buenos Aires, a hotel and *asado* restaurant in Mendoza, and directions for finding Eva Duarte's tomb in the Recoleta Cemetery.

"Oh, by the way," he said, as if digging a minor detail from the back of his mind, "I have a good friend in Buenos Aires, Robert Cox, whom I think you would like to meet. He is editor of the *Buenos Aires Herald*, the English language daily."[3]

"Absolutely," I replied, thinking of the stimulating evening conversations I enjoyed with Bill and his wife Rosie. Maybe I would meet other new friends. "He needs a part for his printing press, which he can't get in Argentina. Would you mind taking it to him for me?"

"I'd be glad to."

The Argentine military had seized political power in 1976 and established a dictatorship that lasted until 1983. Peronists and presumed leftists were captured, tortured, and murdered by the thousands, their bodies thrown into the ocean or otherwise "disappeared" in the Dirty War. Bill didn't tell me this part of the story. When he gave me the part for the printing

---

3. https://en.wikipedia.org/wiki/Buenos_Aires_Herald.

press, he did casually mention that it might be a good idea if customs officers didn't find it. "The piece" was unboxed, un-labeled, shiny silver, the size of a book and weighed a pound or two. I slipped it into my bag between two T-shirts.

When I arrived at Bill's recommended hotel, I told the desk clerk that the friend who had recommended the hotel was a newspaper reporter (*periodista*). He called the manager, who told me that the room I had reserved was not available. He recommended another nearby hotel. In case the manager had called to warn the second hotel, I chose a third.

I called Robert Cox and arranged to take "the piece" to his apartment. There I met him and his wife. We conversed briefly just inside his closed front door. This was contraband exchange, not social intercourse. Smiling, yes. Sitting, drink-ing tea, conversing, no. Within five minutes , I had given him "the piece" and left for my walk through La Recoleta. I later learned that the *Buenos Aires Herald* had been the only news-paper that told the stories of the *desaparecidos*. Robert Cox had been jailed, his family threatened, and his wife almost kidnapped. They left Argentina in 1979.

Maybe "the piece" helped him.

Angel Falls (Salto Angel)

In 1979 I visited *La Casona* (President's residence) in Cara-cas. Horseback trails, bowling alley, dining hall, parking lot for skateboarding—everything teenage kids could want. Lara

78

13 , Darrell 15, and I then drove a rental car to Valencia, Mérida, and Pico Bolívar.

Venezuelan militia at highway checkpoints paid no attention to me—only to Lara. They had never seen a blonde, blue-eyed beauty in real life, only on TV.

That same year, Darrell and I flew to Canaima, Venezuela, from Caracas with Rafael Cortez. The Avensa Boeing 727 buzzed Angel Falls, thrilling Rafael and me, terrorizing Darrell.

To reach the falls from Canaima we used an 18-foot fishing boat with our Russian guide, Anatoly Pochesob, an outboard motor, two crew, plus Darrell, Rafael, and me. During our excursion up Rio Carrao to the base of the falls, Anatoly had us beach the boat to fish for dinner using chicken necks for bait. Although Darrell and the crew were experienced fisherman, they had no luck. We arrived at our destination, Isla Orquídea, at the base of the falls. The fully occupied campground had space for a dozen visitors and no latrines. Anatoly cooked our bait, the chicken necks, for dinner.

Angel Falls is the world's tallest uninterrupted waterfall, 3,212 feet. The next morning we awoke and climbed 1,000 feet to the first overlook, where the falling spray, a river at the top of the tepui, had over centuries carved a beautiful swimming bowl below.

On the boat trip back to Canaima, we stopped to visit a hermit on an island. He was a "psychologist" who had fled

Germany in 1947 and wore only an army blanket wrapped around his shoulders.

Twenty-five years later I returned to Angel Falls with 14-year-old Keith. The legendary Anatoly had died, but an island in the national park had been named in his honor. Isla Orquídea was now crammed with over a hundred campers. Infrastructure was frozen in time and human waste. There were still no latrines.

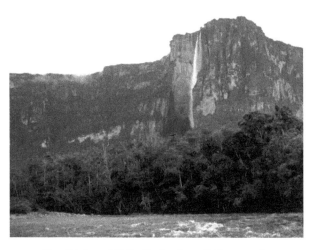

Fig. 15. Angel Falls (Salto Angel), Venezuela.

Buzzards, Rats, and *Los Llaneros*

In 1993 Magda, Keith, and I flew to Los Llanos south of Caracas with Armando Godoy in his Beechcraft Bonanza "35 Papa." Despite skilled laser surgery by *La Eminencia*, Armando relied for visual cues on his wife, Aloma, the co-pilot.

As we were climbing to cruising altitude, I spotted buzzards at 12 o'clock. "How do you say buzzard in Spanish?" I asked Magda. "I don't remember," she replied.

The birds grew larger. Still at 12 o'clock. "*Buitres*!" shouted the co-pilot, and Armando went into a steep dive. "That's it," said Magda. "*Buitres*." Keith held tightly to her, reminding me of Darrell's reaction buzzing Angel Falls.

Los Llanos is an extensive ecoregion of subtropical grasslands, savannas, and wetlands that extends from the Orinoco River in the east into Colombia in the west. Cattle ranching is the primary economic activity. *Los llaneros* in Venezuela are *los gauchos* of the pampas in Argentina and Uruguay, *los vaqueros* of Mexico, and the cowboys of Texas.

We stayed in Armando's thatched-roof cabin on land carved from the jungle. The uncarved jungle surrounding his cabin was inhabited by several groups of Venezuelan red howler monkeys, small but clamorous. They serenaded us at dawn with their namesake operatic roaring, howling chorus as they leapt from branch to branch through the trees. After the morning chorus ended, the only noise in our cabin was the scratching of rats scurrying through the thatch roof. We did not encounter the famous king-size jaguars, which are nocturnal.

Before we left Caracas, Armando had shown me a picture of Bonanza "35 Papa" on the cover of the latest aviation magazine. "You must be proud," I said. He nodded, put the magazine in the trunk of his car, and we left for the airport.

After our return flight two days later, Armando brought the magazine from the trunk. The lead article described a defect in the Bonanza, the plane that had just carried us to jungle and back, that lets the V-tail fall off unexpectedly. The plane then drops like a rock expectedly. I later learned that some called the Bonanza a "Doctor Killer."

Cuenca

In 1989 I was guest of honor at the Ecuadorian congress in Cuenca, the third-largest city in Ecuador. The airline that was to fly me to Cuenca from Guayaquil went out of business a week before my flight, and there were no others available. I rented a car at sea level in Guayaquil to make the 120-mile drive alone, starting in mid-afternoon.

Cuenca is high in the Andes, about 8,400 feet. The road was challenging—hard gravel, curving, no lane or edge markings. There were no maps, no signs for road hazards, directions, or destinations. Nevertheless, the first hour, crossing the coastal plain toward the east, was easy. The ascent into the Andes the second hour taught me what happens when cold, dry mountain air hits hot, humid sea level air from the equator—fog, lots of dense fog.

After I had ascended a thousand feet into the Andes, the road and other vehicles disappeared into the clouds. For the next hour I drove at 20 miles per hour or less on a curving, gravel mountain road with 30-foot visibility. As I reached the plateau, fog cleared enough for me to make out a fork in the road, a fork without a sign. I knew that Quito was to the north, so I turned south. The fog cleared, and I arrived safely in Cuenca after the third hour.

In addition to the Ecuadorian Congress of Ophthalmology, Cuenca was hosting the Second Biennial Congress of Latin American art, a magic combination for me. I spent more time in art than ophthalmology that week. The painting I purchased—a six-foot by six-foot abstract oil by Pablo Barriga—I stored in a Guayaquil bank until an Ecuadorian commercial pilot coming to Miami for consultation offered to bring it to me with the cargo. After the meeting, I returned the rental car in Cuenca and rode to Guayaquil with a colleague who lived in that city.

Miami Vice

From 1970 through 1990, a cocaine-fueled drug war was ongoing in Miami and Latin America—my working territory.

In 1980 I was driven on a tour of the countryside around Santa Cruz, Bolivia.

"Where do you think all the workers are?" asked my host.

"Moved to the city?" I guessed.

"Nope. They all left to work cocaine. Mechanics, carpenters, truck drivers, shop keepers. They deserted every village."

A few years later in Lima, I was invited by my host to visit an artist's studio. The "artist" turned out to be an entrepreneur, who said she owned a pesticide plant. "Do you have cockroaches in Miami?" she asked. "I have a treatment that eliminates them permanently. Here is a sample." She handed me a small plastic bag of white powder as she left me at my Lima hotel.

While packing that night for my return flight home, I dumped the plastic bag into the garbage. At the airport the next day, two customs officers took me into an olive drab, windowless interrogation room. My checked bag was brought into the room and searched. One officer emptied my pockets, shoes, and carry-on, then patted me down. I didn't know why the powder was planted, how I had been targeted, or what was really going on. I simply boarded my plane and returned to Miami. Not until later did I realize that I had been a decoy. An American professor caught with a plastic bag of cocaine would have brought every customs officer in the Lima airport to the interrogation room. A golden opportunity for a mule with a colon full of cocaine-loaded condoms to board the plane undetected.

Following Henry Kissinger

My most memorable art adventure was a visit one evening in 1985 to Carlos and Fani Bracher's home in Ouro Preto, Brazil.[4]

Ouro Preto is the heart of the 17th- and 18th-century Brazilian Gold Rush and the former capital of the mining state, Minas Gerais. Much of the colonial wealth generated in the gold mines was kept in Ouro Preto, legally and otherwise. A popular expression, "*santo do pau oco*," probably originated in this era, referring to a saint carved with a hollow center that contained contraband gold to evade Portugal's tax on precious metals from Brazil. Ouro Preto's colonial wealth is manifest today in the magnificent Portuguese Baroque colonial architecture, the basis for Ouro Preto' designation as a UNESCO World Heritage site. A perfect home for one of Brazil's great landscape artists, Carlos Bracher.

Carlos is a gentle, unassuming man my age with Van Dyke beard, delicate hands, and long light brown hair that looks meant to be blowing in the breeze.

For an hour-and-a-half, until about midnight, we sat in his living room, drinking coffee and chatting. Then, although his preferred genre was landscape, he asked to paint my portrait.

"Magda is so beautiful," I said. "Wouldn't you rather paint her?"

---

4. https://en.wikipedia.org/wiki/Ouro_Preto.

"No, I prefer you," Carlos replied, "I've only painted one other American—Henry Kissinger."

He set up his easel and brushes, changed the lights, and turned on the stereo with a selection from ABBA to Bach to Beatles to the end of the musical alphabet. Sitting in front of me, he underwent a mystical transformation to a completely different person. Intensely focused on his subject, mixing and dipping colors on the palette, swiping and slashing brushes on canvas, glancing at my face, energetically recreating on canvas, as portrait artists do, the essence of the person who was now his friend.

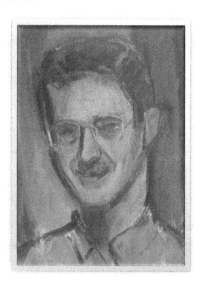

Fig. 16a. 1985 portrait by Carlos Bracher in Ouro Preto, Brazil. "The only other American I ever painted is Henry Kissinger."

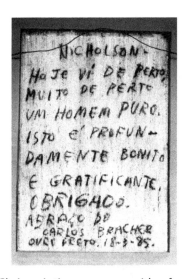

Fig. 16b. Inscription on reverse side of portrait.

In 1989, at the Pan American Congress of Ophthalmology, I visited Bracher's 30-year retrospective exhibition at the National Museum in Rio. To experience the whole trajectory of his work four years after he had painted my portrait in his living room was a humbling experience.[5]

El Maracanazo[6]

A tiny Spanish suffix has a big meaning: "-azo." This suffix is an augmentative attached to a noun to increase its size, importance, effect, or force. In Cuban Miami, the most common application is *Cubanazo*, or *Cubanaza*, which refers to

---

5. https://ateliecasabracher.com/
6. https://en.wikipedia.org/wiki/El_Maracanazo

a person who is *very Cuban*—someone who engages in loud conversations spoken in an "s"-less dialect (*puma* instead of *la espuma*), is extroverted, of generous body proportions, musically and rhythmically inclined, and has a dress style divorced from any accepted couture.

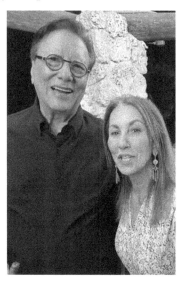

Fig. 17. Two Proud *Cubanazos*. Arturo Sandoval, Cuban-American jazz trumpeter, pianist, and composer raised in Hialeah, winner of multiple Grammys and an Emmy award, plus the Presidential Medal of Freedom, with his omnipresent Cuban cigar and a devoted fan, my wife Sarita, at a Sandoval jazz concert 2022.

Maracanazo applies the "-azo" suffix to the Rio soccer stadium Maracanã. It indicates that something big, significant, scandalous, offensive, illegal, violent, or all, occurred there.

I attended the 1989 Maracanazo with my chief, Edward Norton, who was 67 at the time. At the Pan American Congress of Ophthalmology in Rio, I made him a proposal: "Ed, I know that you have always been a sports fan, particularly for baseball, since your father played semi-pro ball in Massachusetts. While we are here, the Brazilian National Team will play *futebol* (soccer) against the Chilean National team to see who qualifies for the 1990 World Cup. The game will be next Sunday in Maracanã, capacity about one hundred thousand. I have two tickets and round-trip bus transportation from our hotel. Would you like to go? It will be an experience you'll never forget!" I should not have tacked on that last inducement.

"Of course. I've never been to a professional soccer game. What did you call it?"

"*Futebol*."

We arrived at the stadium an hour before the game and found our seats about 50 feet behind the edge of the overhanging deck above. At first, I was disappointed that our tickets were behind the better view from the edge of our deck. However, when the game started, and spectators on the deck above began pouring cups of beer and other clear golden liquids over the edge onto spectators in the first rows of our deck, I was more satisfied with my seat selection.

After the scoreless first period, Ed had to urinate. Fortunately, I accompanied him. The men's room turned out to be a long rectangular open concrete trough, lined with men peeing on both sides. This was my first experience as a bodyguard. I stood behind him, determined to keep this gray-haired, somewhat wobbly, world leader of ophthalmology from being pushed into the trough. When Maracanã was first built, it had no bathrooms at all. So, I guess this was an improvement. We returned safe and dry to our seats for the second period, when the game earned its Chilean name, *El Maracanazo*.

A Brazilian goal in the 47th minute put Brazil ahead 1–0. In the 67th minute, a firecracker or flare exploded a few feet in front of the Chilean goalkeeper, Roberto Rojas, who began bleeding profusely from his face and fell to the ground. Pandemonium erupted. Chilean players left the field in protest. One of the Chilean players insulted Brazilian fans by grabbing his genitals, which were covered by his soccer shorts. Chilean fans immortalized the gesture as "el Pato Yáñez" (Yáñez's duck) to honor the player who perfected it.[7]

Armed soldiers cordoned off the field to protect players and officials from angry fans streaming down from the first terrace of seats. Officials canceled the game pending further investigation.

---

7. https://www.youtube.com/watch?v=37rXg6SZ2-k

"Well, Ed, what did you think?" I asked on the bus to our hotel.

"Who won?" he wondered.

"We'll find out in the next few days, I imagine. At least there was no war".

"War?"

"Twenty years ago, El Salvador defeated Honduras three to two to qualify for the 1970 World Cup. El Salvador broke diplomatic relations and attacked Honduras a few days later, resulting in the 'Soccer War.'"[8]

The Chilean goalkeeper, Rojas, later confessed that he had slashed his own face with a concealed razor blade to simulate an attack by Brazilian fans. Somehow, Chileans had recruited a 24-year-old Brazilian model, Rosenery Mello do Nascimento, to throw the flare toward Rojas from the Brazilian spectator section. She was crowned the "Firecracker of Maracanã" and featured on the cover of *Playboy*.

FIFA, the international governing World Cup body, declared Brazil the victor by a score of 2–0, defeating Chile's brazen attempt to steal a spot in World Cup competition.

Gipuzkoa

San Sebastian (Donostia) was our favorite city in Iberia, and we returned several times.

---

8. https://en.wikipedia.org/wiki/Football_War

In 1991 after a guest lecture, as I was driving from the Miramar Palace parking lot onto a four-lane undivided highway, I apparently merged like a Miamian. The driver behind me veered into the left lane, rolled down the passenger window, and shouted as he passed: "*TU ESPAÑOL.*" It was the worst insult he could muster—"YOU SPANIARD." You see, San Sebastian is in Gipuzkoa (Basque Country), where Spaniards are considered a tribe of ignorant savages. I had obviously merged like a Madrileño rather than a Miamian.

In 2006 we drove west from San Sebastian in the hills above the *Golfo de Vizcaya* on a curving, two-lane concrete road with no shoulder on its bayside edge. I gave an oncoming car too much room and my right rear wheel slipped off the edge of the road. I stopped, shifted into reverse, lightly pressed the gas, and my right front wheel slipped off the edge. With both right wheels off the edge of the road, the car tilted a few degrees downhill, rocking gently. I opened the driver's door and stood with my weight inside the car to keep it from rolling down the mountainside, while Magda gingerly edged across to my side. We got out safely.

Just uphill was a memorial cross for another driver who hadn't been so lucky.

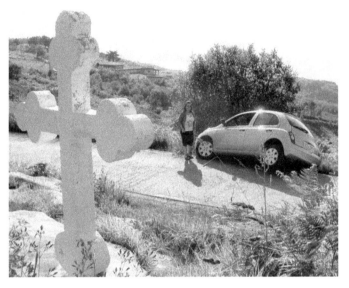

Fig. 18a. 2006. Gipuzcoa. Magda emerged safely from the rental car, which leans ready to plunge into Golfo de Vizcaya.

Within 20 minutes, five cars and two bicycles had stopped to help. Eighteen adults, a toddler, and a dog.

"Can you call a tow truck?" I asked. They walked around the car.

"No hace falta—somos Vascos." Not necessary—we're Basques. They walked around again, exchanged a few words, took their positions, and lifted the car onto the road.

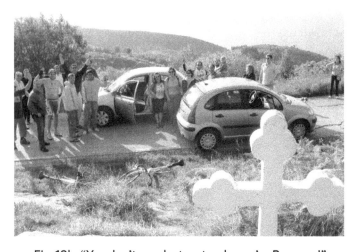

Fig.18b. "You don't need a tow truck—we're Basques!"

Coda

In 1994 I was at the annual Peruvian Congress of Ophthalmology. The other guest of honor was one of the 20th century's most revered leaders, Dr. Charles Schepens (1912–2006)—Belgian resistance fighter against the Nazis in WW II, inventor of the key to successful retinal detachment surgery, founder of The Retina Foundation in Boston—the list goes on. He was the elder statesman of world ophthalmology in 1994. Dr. Schepens, his wife, Cette, and I were taken on a private tour of the Larco Museum of Erotic Art. With Dr. Charles Schepens, a living legend, I spent the afternoon

94

perusing and discussing Peruvian pre-Columbian erotic pottery.

In 1996 a patient was referred from Costa Rica, Óscar Arias Sánchez. Arias, a previous president of Costa Rica, had won the Nobel Peace Prize in1987 for his plan to end years of civil wars in Central America. During his examination in my office, I resisted the temptation to ask President Arias for details about Costa Rican pre-Columbian erotic pottery.

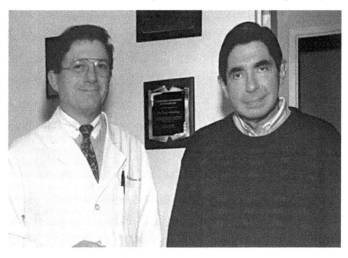

Fig. 19. 1996. Patient Óscar Arias Sánchez, former president of Costa Rica and Nobel Peace laureate in 1987.

Chapter 13

Robert

A few years after I retired, my brother Robert, 14 years my junior, died at age 46.

When he was only three years old, Robert splashed ink over the presentation poster for my Tennessee state high school science fair entry. I reacted with kindness and equanimity. I simply started preparing the poster again from scratch. It was an excellent lesson that I wish I had always kept in mind.

When I left for Stanford, Robert was four, and we parted for years. I became an outside observer of his life.

Robert went to Andover prep in Massachusetts. In 1970 while he was at Andover, Robert visited us in Watertown. He and I saw the first run of the movie *M*A*S*H*, and he introduced me to Cat Stevens (Yusuf). He then went to Stanford for one year and later enrolled at Rhodes College in Memphis, where he graduated Phi Beta Kappa with an A.B. in psychology. He then received his Ph.D. at the University of Texas at Austin.

Between Stanford and Rhodes, Magda and I took Robert and his girlfriend "K" on a bareboat charter in the Virgin Islands. Robert was an incompetent first-time sailor, trapping his glove in the halyard as he hoisted the main, shouting more in fear than pain. Thereafter, we called our 41-foot Morgan ketch *Expectoration* instead of *Expectation*.

When we tried to anchor at a mooring buoy at the Bitter End Yacht Club in Virgin Gorda, I approached the buoy several times with Robert leaning over the bow, unable to catch the mooring buoy with the grappling hook. Finally, K shouted in her Tennessee twang, "Robert. Quit battin' that orange ball and stop the boat! Magda and I want to wash our hair."

A cocktail crowd of yachtsmen gathered on the Bitter End dock to watch the ball-batting, followed by the garbage boat motoring out to attach our boat to the mooring buoy. Magda and K returned from the Bitter End shower after their critical hair wash while I was below taking a nap. I awakened to a faint female voice: "Robert ... Robert ... the dinghy ... the dinghy." I leapt out of the bunk and raced to the deck.

Our now-coiffed deckhands had not secured the dinghy, which floated peacefully toward Prickly Pear Island. I dove overboard, swam to the dinghy, and brought it back to *Expectoration*. The cocktail crowd had moved inside to dinner, not realizing that they had missed Act Three. Magda and K had been paralyzed on deck by their two-dollar showers and first hair wash in a week.

Robert and K married, had two precious daughters, and moved to Jackson MS, where Robert completed his postgraduate training. He became an expert in forensic psychological assessment, including competency to stand trial. He was then welcomed to the faculty of the University of Tulsa, where he began a distinguished professional career. Their marriage, however, lasted only a few years. Robert had two sons afterward.

He called me in early 2000 from the hospital, suffering from pneumonia. I agreed to come help him at home in Tulsa after he was discharged. Buying groceries, preparing meals, keeping doctors' appointments, and loving my baby brother were my main duties. The two-week recovery period gave us our first and last opportunity to have long, personal, uninterrupted conversations.

Six months later he died.

I had been on the phone with him from Miami two days before, listening to his labored breathing and description of symptoms that let me know he had severe heart failure. I recommended that he seek immediate help at the emergency room. He did and was admitted to the hospital.

Although he was still in heart failure and could hardly breathe, his doctor from the pneumonia episode six months earlier ordered an emergency bone marrow aspiration.

The hematologist arrived, positioned Robert on his back, as was the standard protocol, and began to perform an iliac bone marrow aspiration. Robert was suffocating. Positioned flat on his back, the pulmonary edema from his heart failure drowned him, and he died.

Mom, Janet, and I arrived in Tulsa soon after Robert's death. Mom handled funeral arrangements, Janet and I concentrated on cleaning the house and selling his few belongings to start a trust account for his four children. During our time in Tulsa, I received a copy of his hospital medical record from the mother of his two sons.

Buried in the lab results from his pneumonia hospitalization was a urinalysis. Bence-Jones protein had been detected in the urine, evidence that was ignored or missed at the time. Robert's primary underlying disease was multiple myeloma, a blood cancer composed of plasma cells in the blood and bone marrow. Myeloma frequently causes heart failure.

The internist who had rushed to order the bone marrow aspiration was trying to cover his incompetence, to hide having missed the diagnosis, a blinking red light in Robert's urinalysis six months earlier.

What should I do?

The decision was easy.

I found the best plaintiff's malpractice lawyer in Tulsa, presented my evidence, and he took the case. A few months later he won a settlement from the involved doctor, hospital, and insurance companies. The four children had enough money in their trust funds to pay for college.

Chapter 14

My Mother's Life

In September, 2005, during my monthly visit to Memphis, Mom and I set up a series of interviews to give succeeding generations some recollections of her life. We had four interview conversations using a digital tape recorder at her dining-room table. It had been almost six years since Dad's death. Mom was 90 years old, sharp and lively as ever. Each evening before the next day's performance, we would discuss the proposed topics—times, places, people, and events. I wrote an outline. She needed no outline, notes, journal, or computer search. An accomplished actor, debate winner, and sought-after public speaker, she was in her element.

I was a rookie interviewer enjoying a few relaxed and charming hours with my mother.

For clarity and relevance in this chapter, I abridged the conversations from typed transcripts.

I sent copies of the unabridged recordings to Janet and each of Mother's grandchildren.

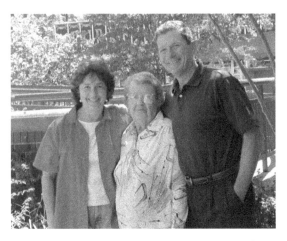

Fig. 20. Memphis, 2004. Janet, Rosemary, and Don.

Interview 1: 1916–1945

Don:

It's September 30, 2005. This will be the first in a series of interviews with Rosemary Nicholson—Mom, Mama Nick—to get some memories of her long, loving life. Today, we're going to talk about her memories of those years through the end of WWII. Mom?

Rosemary:

I was born in Pleasanton, Kansas, and moved to Oklahoma City, where we bought a house. I remember it was green wash, not a paint, and it had a front porch with two brick columns at the side and two more brick columns down by the steps. I said, "This house has chimneys all over it!" Two bedrooms and a sleeping porch.

I wanted so badly to go to school. I entered kindergarten at age four. In grade school I met a wonderful mix of children. Oklahoma City's Home for Children, for orphans and children who needed a foster home, was two blocks from my school, Wilson Elementary. Across the street in the other direction was the wealthiest area in town.

Don:

Can you tell me about your family—mother, father, brother?

Rosemary:

I had a mother that I adored and a father who had his alcohol problems, but you couldn't help adoring him. He had a wonderful personality and a good reputation with everyone except us. I didn't feel any neglect or anything of the sort, though I remember seeing him once trying to choke my mother. We were in his little clothing store in downtown Oklahoma City. A tailor was right there but would not come out to help her. His job depended on minding his own business, I guess. After my mother came to, she, my brother, and I rode home on the streetcar. The other similar incident I remember was that once he held a knife to her throat. Both of those were drunken adventures, and he had so many nice times. Sometimes he could go a year without a drink, but if he was offered a drink, he was gone. Once his employer at the Oklahoma Publishing Company hired a man to go with him as he sold advertisements to try to keep him straight.

Don:

His name was Edgar Taylor?

Rosemary:

Edgar Marion Taylor. My brother, two years older than I, was Edward, my mother's father's name. My mother's name was Lena Muenchmeyer. Her father was German, her mother English. My grandfather was tall and wiry, his wife little and plump. They lived in Bartlesville, 150 miles north of Oklahoma City. I knew him better in his old age. Saturday night my grandmother would say, "Papa … Papa … it's time to take your bath." He'd scoot down a little in his chair as if he were disappearing. She'd repeat a bit louder, "Papa, come on."

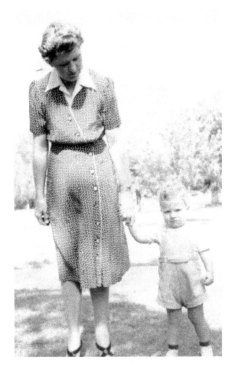

Fig. 21. 1942. My grandmother, Lena Muenchmeyer Taylor, and the author.

Don:

Let's talk about junior high and high school.

Rosemary:

I lived 12 blocks from the junior high school, so I walked. One winter it was snowing hard. About two blocks from our home, a big football player picked me up and carried me along the streetcar tracks the rest of the way to school. Usually, it was fine just to walk.

In seventh grade I began to try out for debate. The boys' team had Johnny Walbert. He was smart, but he could not say the word "statistics." We tried in rebuttal or whenever we could, to get him to say that. It would always come out "stah-*stis*-tics."

I also started trying out for plays, one each year. Miss Blaine Tucker, our drama teacher, was wonderful. At auditions I won the lead in every play except one. That one went to a friend of mine, Jane Lyons. When she had the lead in that one, the director gave me the part of Lallie Joy, who had a speech like an oration. When I finished, the whole audience clapped and clapped. Thrilled me to death.

I never remember in junior or senior high my father coming to see even one of my performances. How I would have loved it, but I didn't seem to miss it then. A next-door neighbor, Mrs. Dodson, would go with Mother, and we had a good time. Somehow, it didn't seem to affect me or make me long for him to be there.

After junior high, I went to Classen High School, about the same distance from our house in a different direction. I continued to enjoy dramatics. The year that I went to Classen High, my drama coach was transferred to that same school. So, I had the same instructor for six years! I just loved her. Miss Tucker had a walk that kept her little elbows tucked in against her body. I tried to imitate it but couldn't.

My junior year of high school, I had to move with my mother to Bartlesville to live with my grandmother and grandfather. We weren't able to stay in our home that year; Mother rented her house for $35 a month.

I had a good opportunity to learn which uncomfortable situation I should feel responsible for and which I should not. Two doors from me on the corner was a girl in my same grade, Virginia Lee. Sometimes she let me visit her house after school. She lived with her grandparents who drank, but less than her mother did. Virginia's grandfather would often be passed out on the floor at the front door. She'd merely say, "You'll have to step over my grandfather," and not miss a beat. That circumstance did not upset her, and I knew I could do the same.

That was the summer of Grandpa Muenchmyers's Saturday night disappearing act. Grandfather Muenchmeyer told me that with his fortune from oil royalties on his land, Chief Bacon Rind (1860–1932) built a showplace mansion with a separate room for his favorite horse. He also kept a grand piano under the branches of a large elm tree in his yard. In later years I'd visit my grandmother in the summertime. Now that my children and grandchildren have traveled so much, I tell them, "Well, I got to go to my grandmother's from Oklahoma City to Bartlesville and spend a whole week in the summer."

The summer before my Bartlesville year I met Howard at a Sunday evening Methodist Youth Fellowship program, which I was leading. Two men had come into the room, the first grown men that had ever looked at me. They sat on the front row and stared right through me. I made the mistake of asking, "Is there anything anyone wants to sing?" The best friend sitting next to Howard, Jack Fleming, said, "Let's sing something bloody—'Onward Christian Soldiers.'"

Afterward, Howard walked down the stairs with me to learn my name and address. Much as I would like to have given them to him, I did not. He called a friend who lived a block from me and got the information from him. He told Howard, "She'll be at the church next Wednesday night for a meeting." Howard came to the meeting. Then he got into the car that was taking me home with another boy and girl. When the driver stopped at my house, Howard said, "I'll just get out with her."

"Oh no, you won't," the driver-father warned. He took Howard to his own home. That summer Howard and I went out several times. He was driving a truck for

Camp Grocery, a rickety delivery truck without a passenger door. I felt as if I was going to fall out any minute, but I didn't dare mention it. We'd go to a drive-in restaurant, and each eat a nickel hamburger. Then he'd head back to his deliveries and other work.

He graduated two years before me and had won the outstanding boy graduate award at Classen High. I did not know that at the time. I won the outstanding girl graduate award two years after Howard's award. When I won the award, Mrs. Nicholson, Howard's mother, called my mother to congratulate her. I told Mother, "She didn't call to congratulate. She called to make sure we knew that Howard had won the same award." I loved when that happened!

The next year, after my sixteenth birthday, was the year that I had to go to Bartlesville. I kept expecting to hear from Howard. I wrote to him once, and he wrote to me once. Finally, I got my mother to stare south toward Oklahoma City and thumb her nose at Howard. I'm sure she didn't care for that, but I thought that's what he deserved.

Don:

When you graduated from high school, didn't you have a scholarship arranged to go to college?

Rosemary:

Oh, yes. Miss Tucker, my wonderful drama teacher had taken the time, effort, and lying or telling the truth to arrange a four-year scholarship for me at Judson College, Alabama. I'd never seen the school, but it must have been good in drama, because my teacher had graduated from there. I was all set to go. I had my grip packed and my picture on the society page of the *Daily Oklahoman* with two friends.

My dad said he thought he could make it sober if I stayed at home, and that's all it took. I not only didn't go, but I did not thank Miss Tucker for all she must have put into it. It just didn't enter my head that it shouldn't be my right because I had earned it.

I took a course in shorthand that uses regular letters, and I knew that pretty well. I began to look for a job to pay for tuition at Oklahoma City University the next year, when I would be 17. OCU was fairly near my house, and I could probably be accepted.

My jobs in the Great Depression were WPA jobs. I had two jobs that each paid $15 a month. You weren't supposed have more than one, but I didn't let either of my teacher–employers know. I had to go to one teacher, see if she needed me to write letters, then go to the other and ask if he needed any typing. If one did, I would walk across the street to the journalism department, type the letter, and take it back.

In college that year, in addition to all the required courses, I took accounting. There was a rich boy in our class who couldn't get it, so the family hired me as his accounting tutor. At times I even got to ride in his convertible. I enjoyed anything with mathematics, so bookkeeping came easily for me. I had only the one year of college at OCU.

In 1933 I got a job through the father of a friend of mine at Travelers Insurance Company. I worked there for several years and loved it. When Howard and I decided to get married, the company made me quit. A married woman could not work, because it would take the job from a man. When I had to quit Travelers, I got another job in the same building. It was as much money, but not as nice. In 1936 Howard and I married, and the company had a lovely shower for me. I didn't write a thank you note to any of the guests, because I saw them every day at work. That's how little I knew about social graces.

I had one other job, at Anderson Pritchard Oil Company, that I'd like to mention. The interviewer asked: "Do you know the Dewey Decimal System?" I said, "Yes."

The only thing I knew about it was that libraries use the system to organize books. I thought I could find out what it was at the public library. Turns out, you can't, because it's a little more complicated than that. Nevertheless, I set about rearranging all the oil company files. I'm sure they haven't found some of those files yet in the Rosemary–Dewey Decimal System.

Don:

At one of those jobs, I remember, the boss used to chase you around the desk

Rosemary:

After I left the Travelers Insurance Company, my new boss, about 55, claimed that I looked like his young lover years before and started chasing me around the desk. I would figure out a way to avoid him—and always did. When his wife came to the office to see him for some reason, I would put a fresh piece of paper in my typewriter and type "now is the time for all good men to come to the aid of their country," the training exercise typists practice to perfection.

Don:

Over and over and over again ...

Rosemary:

Yeah, to show both of them how fast I typed.

Howard and I decided that we wanted to have a baby the next year, our fifth year of marriage. I was so excited I could have run for home anytime!

As soon as I knew I was pregnant, I was thrilled to death, but it boggled my mind to think of all the responsibilities. So anyway, we were having happy times. Howard would come in off the road after five days and say, "Where are we going tonight?"

Don:

What sorts of things did you like to do?

Rosemary:

We loved to be with our good friends in our homes, or at the Variety Club.

I've often regretted never thanking Lena or Gaga for staying with you. I knew either of them had to be thrilled and grateful for the chance. Of course, I was thrilled to get away!

Within six months after we married, my dad was hospitalized in Tulsa, then had a stroke.

Don:

After that you and Dad moved back into Lena's house?

Rosemary:

We thought we could help take care of him. He was careless with cigarettes, and there was always a mess around his wheelchair.

Before the stroke, he had been so smart. When I was a secretary working at the Oklahoma Publishing Company, he had one room of wordsmiths and one room of artists.

He and his people put together the advertisements, publicity, and graphics for all the publications. He was head of the department.

By 1939 the house was a disaster; my dad was getting angrier and messier. Mother had him sent to Central State Hospital in Norman, which specialized in chronic neurological problems.

Don:

WWII was declared at the end of 1941. What happened then?

Rosemary:

We were optimistic that Howard would miss the draft. He was 29 years old, still eligible, but with one child and another on the way. We thought the odds were in his favor.

Without knowing it, I put his draft notice on the 1943 Christmas tree. When he read the notice and I saw the look on his face, I knew that he was going overseas. I was pregnant with Janet, and we spent the remaining eight months together as much as possible.

The Army Air Force assigned him to active duty and departure for the Pacific. Howard protested, "I haven't even had my basic training yet."

The Army Air Force said, "Do you think you need it?"

He replied, "I know I do."

They assigned him to another outfit that went to Texas for basic training. He had to jump over obstacles that were difficult for 20-year-olds. Howard held up well, but when he returned in 1944, he was assigned for departure to California. The unit that left without basic training never went to war.

Howard called from California and said the wives of some of his buddies were coming. Could I try? At that time, we had a baby girl less than two months old, and you, three and-a-half years old. I left Janet with the Loys, but the only place I could find for you was a Catholic nursery.

Don:

Orphanage.

Rosemary:

Orphanage was it?

Don:

Definitely.

Rosemary:

You were absolutely miserable ... and I was absolutely happy.

Don:

How did you find Howard? His unit's location was Top Secret. Signs on the walls said, "Loose lips sink ships."

Rosemary:

When I began to inquire in California, every older person told me, "I don't know" or "I can't tell you." I finally found a young person with a sparkle in her eye, who found out where his outfit was.

Don:

In Riverside.

Rosemary:

Riverside, California. We rented a charming little cabin, called Winken, Blinken, and Nod, at a hotel called The Land of Tomorrow. We had one wonderful week together. But remember, I was gone for three weeks—one whole week for travel by train each way.

During that wonderful week I spent with Howard, I forgot that I had a three-and-a-half-year-old at home who was missing his regular surroundings. Mrs. Dodson, the next-door neighbor, volunteered to help. She and Lena took Don from the orphanage to their homes. Mrs. Dodson took care of you during the daytime, and Lena cared for you after she finished her day's office work. I had left three-month-old Janet with two couples. They shared her and kept telling me how wonderful it was to hear Janet laughing at the rustling trees in their yards.

Don:

How long was Dad on Saipan?

Rosemary:

His was the first group to leave for Saipan to prepare for arrival of the B-29s, so they could begin to bomb Japan immediately. He was there about 18 months.

Don:

What did you do while he was overseas?

Rosemary:

I always worked. I traveled for research companies, like Jay Walter Thompson out of Chicago or New York. Another one was convenient to Mrs. Nicholson's house. I'd leave you and Janet with her. Janet would get all the pots from under the sink and spread them all over the kitchen floor. I never put them back where they belonged when I arrived after work. I thought Mrs. Nicholson was lucky to be able to care of you.

On one job I measured the galvanized metal that a person had on this property, usually a farm. "How long do you expect this washtub to last?" Was a typical question.

At a well-cared-for house the owner look at me like, "*What a silly question*. It lasts forever." At a run-down house, the answer was, "Oh, 'bout a year."

Don:

Is there any more you would like to tell us about the sleeping porch?

Rosemary:

In wintertime, we would sleep there with the tarpaulin curtains rolled down. Mother would heat a brick in the oven, wrap it in a towel, and put it down by Dad's feet and mine. It felt wonderful!

I would get in bed with my dad, and he would tell me a story that always wound up with a little female heroine named Rosemary. I was so excited when he told me a story that ended with Rosemary! I never got used to it. It was always a new experience.

Later, during the war, when the children and I lived with my mother, we were surrounded by neighbors who treated you as one of their own. You didn't go to their homes much, but they always knew where he was. Once the man across the street, Mr. Murphy, came over to tell me, "Your son in the front yard is cold in his playpen!"

Another neighbor, Mary Northway, took me on trips with her to Mexico City, California, and Colorado before you were born. Maybe I thanked her for it—that would be a first for me.

Don:

Mary Northway's husband owned the Ford dealership. He was working all the time, and she had enough money to travel, but she didn't have a companion until she met you.

Rosemary:

> She was a former nurse. Sometimes her foot would swell; she'd find a tight bandage and continue driving. The year you were born, Howard told Mary that he was going to give me a car on the next Mother's Day.
>
> I received his Mother's Day card. It was the same year he had given *his* mother the fare to visit Iowa to see her old home. And he gives me *a card*.
>
> That evening Mary called to ask what I had received for Mother's Day.
>
> "Howard gave me a card," I sighed. "I didn't even open it!" Then I told her what he had given his mother.
>
> "Open the card," she said. Inside the card was the title to the black 1940 Ford coupe that he had bought for me!
>
> Whenever people talk now about belts they use to buckle their children into seats, or airbags to protect their faces, I remember my system. The restraint was my right hand. Grab a leg if the kid starts to fall out.

Interview 2: 1945–1950

Don:

> This will be the second interview with Rosemary Nicholson. Mama Nick—the part of her life that begins at the end of World War II. Rosemary is now 28. Her husband returning from Saipan is 33, and they have two

children—Don, five, and Janet, one and a half. Can you take up where we left off, Mom?

Rosemary:

At that particular time, we could not even find a place to live. The children and I had been staying with Mother on 22nd Street in Oklahoma City. All veterans were guaranteed their pre-war job, so that part was fine. Finally, we decided to move into a tiny house we had bought before the war to rent as an investment.

Then we started getting transfer offers from Paramount to move anywhere in Texas. We chose San Antonio, then Dallas. We found a place on Reverchon Drive, next door to Sebe and Margie Miller, good friends of ours in Paramount. I learned about the house while we were at an annual Paramount picnic. I left the picnic, rented the house, and drove back to watch the Dallas Paramount softball team beat Oklahoma City. The house was an adorable little two bedroom place on a quiet street, with next-door neighbors we already knew

We lived there until we found the house in Highland Park, a two story brick house in excellent condition within two blocks of the elementary school and a small shopping center. It was an elegant part of town convenient to downtown Dallas, where the Paramount office was located.

Don:

> That was the first house you had owned since Oklahoma City. Do you remember how much you paid for it?
>
> Rosemary: I think we bought it for $17,000, then sold it for $21,000 when we were transferred to Memphis a few years later.

Don:

> Those were gypsy years for you. You lived in five different houses during a period of five years, and you were able to remain in the Highland Park house for less than two years. They transferred you in 1951 to Memphis, when Dad was promoted to branch manager.

Rosemary:

> He was in Memphis for 12 years. Those were the glory days for the children because they had a screening every Friday night at the Paramount office. Not only Paramount releases, but any company's new picture. The children were able to invite a guest, as well. That's the longest we'd ever been any one place together.
>
> We found our dream house at 1819 Forrest through the kindness of a neighbor, who called me at our apartment on Tutwiler.
>
> "Rosemary, get over here now! My next-door neighbor died a few day ago and the family is here from out of town."

I said, "I wouldn't think of it when they've just had a death in the family."

The next day she called again and said, "Get over here! The heirs are here, and they're going to sell that house." So, we bought that lovely home—a basement, downstairs living room, three bedrooms and bath upstairs, attic and dilapidated servants' quarters, where Don set up his dissection laboratory in high school.

Our youngest son, Robert, was born soon after we moved into that house. I had left a note on the staircase to tell Janet to go the next-door neighbor's house. The neighbor helped her get ready for school and gave her another note from me. "I've gone to the hospital to get you a Valentine." Robert was born the next day—February 14.

Don:

You mentioned my first anatomy studies. You had a very important role in those.

Rosemary:

I will never forget that. I might forget you, but I won't forget that experience.

I went to the humane shelter each week to get a cat that they had just euthanized to bring it home for you to dissect. By the time you had worked out there a little while, you were putting blue dye in veins and red dye in arteries.

One day I started home with my dead cat in a box in the back seat, and I heard a thump, thump, thump. I didn't look, I didn't say a word. I just turned straight around and went back to the pound. The veterinarian told me it wasn't dead enough. They gave me a completely dead one, and I drove back home. When you started dissecting pig embryos, I would go to the slaughterhouse and wait for a pregnant sow to be slaughtered. The embryos were put in my back seat cardboard box. None ever thumped on the way home.

I think that the reason I loved those years of your working on dead cats and pig embryos so much was because, while we were still living in Dallas, a doctor looked at a paper you had written. It didn't say, "I want to be a doctor when I grow up." It said, "I must be a doctor." So that's all you ever considered doing. That's why having that room out in back and running dead animal deliveries was so dear to me.

Don:

Can you tell me about your memories of Janet, from ages six to 17 in Memphis?

Rosemary:

Well, I remember making clothes for her. She was such a doll. Even when she was old enough to date, I might be putting the zipper in the side of an evening dress while the young man was knocking at the front door. Usually, I did a little better than that.

There was a piano in the house when we bought it. Janet took piano lessons, and one day I reminded her that her recital was that afternoon. I said, "You'd better go practice."

"I know it."

She went to the piano, played "BANG" and said "WHOOPS," and that was her recital practice. We called her the WHOOPS girl for a while afterward.

One day she told me that during a recital she had been in a recycling. I thought she was doing perfectly, but she had forgotten how to end the piece. She was recycling beautifully, playing and playing and playing. I don't know how she ever stopped.

Don:

Your year in Pittsburgh ended in 1963. Dad was 52, you were 48, and you embarked on an entirely new career. Can you tell us about those years owning and managing a drive-in theater?

Rosemary:

We certainly wouldn't have done it had you calculated our ages at the time! It was so much fun to take over a drive-in that had been neglected. Howard got on the loudspeaker one night and said, "No more stale popcorn at the 51 Drive-in Theater." I thought, "Howard! How can you say that? Everybody listening knows the previous owners, the Ellis family."

We didn't worry too much about money because there wasn't much. I would leave after closing and counting, drive to deposit the money, and return home to Janet and Robert.

Howard was working his tail off. I was doing nothing but counting money at night and keeping the records, which I loved. Sailors on the base at Millington Naval Air Station came to the 51 Drive-In, even though they didn't have cars. Howard had installed rows of wooden folding chairs in front of the projection booths, and dozens of sailors walked from the base every night to sit and watch the movie.

When business got better, Howard would exhibit a picture that we knew we could play as a second feature every six months. *Tobacco Road* was one, but the most popular was *Walking Tall* with Joe Don Baker as Sherriff

Bradford Pusser. We could have played *Walking Tall* every month!

Howard went to court to get pictures as quickly as theaters could get them in Memphis. The major chains in Memphis got first-run pictures, and smaller theaters had to wait for the second round. Drive-in theaters had to wait for the third. Howard had the advantage of having worked on both ends of the negotiations, and he won the right to bid for pictures in the first round.

After we'd had the drive-in for several years, Howard decided to twin it. We had to buy the property from the same person who had originally owned the drive-in site. He refused to sell the land. I said to Howard, "Just tell him that we'll have to go back to Dallas and build our twin theater there." The owner decided to sell us the property.

For the first couple of years, we kept the theater open all year, which was a financial disaster in winter, before the invention of in-car heaters. One January night when no one had arrived by show time, Howard called a friend in and asked, "I don't have any customers here tonight. What do I do? Do I start the movie, or do I wait?" The friend told him, "Go to church next Sunday and put an extra nickel in the collection plate."

We learned not to open year round, to avoid the few bad months. During summertime, we had very good business for a little cow town like Millington. A new screen blowing down in a windstorm and an overflowing creek flood were recoverable dips like those that affect all small businesses.

Once Howard hired a company to align our car ramps by the speakers, so that every car would have a perfect view of the screen. Surveyors, engineers, and heavy equipment were all over the place. It cost us a lot of money. Then came the flood that erased all the newly aligned ramps.

I called a friend who had owned theaters in Arkansas: "We spent an awful lot of money to align the parking ramps with the screen. How do you do it?"

She said, "My mom drives the tractor, and I walk in front of her with my left arm down and my right arm straight toward the screen." After the flood, we used the Arkansas Method to realign our ramps.

Don:

The flood and the windstorm weren't the only hardships that you had. Dad was almost 60 years old and had been in the business about eight years. He was still climbing up a ladder to the sign on U.S. Highway 51 to change the feature and the stars every week. One night after the drive-in had closed, about 2:00 a.m., he fell off the sign, about 15 feet onto a hard gravel surface, fracturing his arm, leg, and pelvis. The place was deserted, out in the middle of the country. He was lying on the gravel about 50 yards away from the highway.

Rosemary:

We were lucky that no cars turned around there that night because they frequently did. A policeman came to my door to tell me the news. I quickly put on Howard's overcoat and went out there. I had always been afraid when I was having a baby that I might say something bad. I asked him, "Howard, how long have you been here?" He calmly replied, "Oh, I have called and crawled interminably." He had never used that word since I had known him, but that was what he said. There was no ambulance service in Millington, so a hearse owned by a local Black funeral company carried him to the hospital. He had quite a bit wrong with him, as Don said, with a slow recovery period. He was beginning to have things happen to him that were very frightening at a time in our lives when we wanted more togetherness.

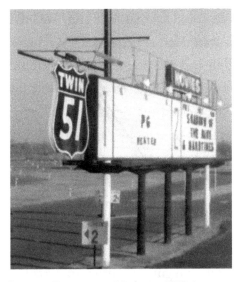

Fig. 22. Millington, Tennessee. Highway 51 Twin marquee, where Dad fell at age 60.

Don:

Speaking of togetherness, Robert was the only child in the house. What was that like?

Rosemary:

It was fun letting Robert grow up in Millington with the freedom of having other friends, and he certainly did have them. Howard was president of the Rotary Club and the Chamber of Commerce. Those activities took evening hours on certain nights, but he made time to do them, run the drive-in, and be a loving father. He was a hard worker, especially when it came to booking the very best pictures he could for that little area. We lived on a street called Howard Place. I pretended it was named for us.

We only had one attempted robbery in all those years. The man was on foot, crossed a cultivated, empty field, and walked toward the ticket booth. I was just getting into my car to come home, and a man's head appeared at the passenger side window. He had a little knife in his hand. I thought, "If I can start this car, I will be a hero." Apparently, I did. I left the money in a cigar box in the car when I jumped out and rushed up to the closest car watching the movie. I tried to shout, but no words came, only sputters and gurgles. I drove to the concession stand and was able to tell the story. After giving the police report, I went home. My money was still in the cigar box.

Among the many good experiences was our constant supply of high quality part-time help. Sailors from the naval air station were eager for extra work, they were educated, and they worked hard.

Don:

You also had at least one high-quality volunteer. When Lara was a teenager, she loved to drive from Florida to be with her grandparents and work odd jobs at the drive-in.

Rosemary:

I will never know whether Lara came because she liked her grandparents, or because she liked to sweep the patio where sailors sat to watch the movie. They had an opportunity to talk with a pretty young girl, and the pretty young girl had the opportunity to talk with handsome young sailors. I'm glad *Officer and a Gentleman* wasn't released until years later!

Every so often Howard hosted a live movie star at the drive-in. Police volunteered to pick them up at the city limits. Not pick them up bodily, but accompany their car, red and blue lights flashing brightly. Howard borrowed a flatbed trailer from a neighboring farmer to serve as the stage. The star could sing, talk, and woo the crowd—a lot of fun. What a wonderful business. Howard had to work and work, but I didn't have to do that.

Don:

Let me ask you about your IRS in-house audit in Millington.

Rosemary:

Until the IRS informed us that an agent was coming to our house to audit our return, I didn't realize that a business with all cash income was almost certain to be subjected to an in-house audit. I set the agent up at our breakfast room table and put our complete box of records on the table. I learned later that you don't do this—it's best to wait for a specific request and then find the item they ask for. Don't show them anything else.

Before the agent arrived we removed everything that didn't belong to the drive-in from the storeroom behind our house. We turned off the automatic telephone answering machine, so the whole time the agent was sitting at the table, I was answering the phone, telling people what was playing that night, and answering their questions. When I wasn't answering calls, I was ironing aprons for employees at the drive in, another new role for me. As he was leaving at noon, the agent said, "If everyone kept records like yours, I'd have an easier job, and they'd have fewer problems." He never came back.

Don:

During those years you also had two grandchildren who lived close by in Memphis. Could you tell us about Tracy and Trip, Janet's children?

Rosemary:

Janet and Jack Leonard divorced when the children were young, and they both lived with her. We were able to help her as best we could.

We had had such fun with Tracy. The next-door neighbors knew that when she was at my house, she could visit them with a little timer in her hand, set to ring in 10 or 15 minutes. Then they sent her home.

One winter night Janet was also staying with us. Tracy got up and crept out the door to visit the neighbors. She walked through the snow alone, barefoot in the middle of the night. She arrived in her little white gown with no timer. The neighbors immediately carried her back to our house. Tracy died in a car accident at age 16.

After Tracy's death we got to spend time with Trip, give him jobs at the drive-in, and foster a loving relationship. One time Trip was earning money by raking leaves in our yard. Oh, he raked and raked, and didn't get through until dark. I looked out the window and saw that he had finished his work and was jumping into his carefully arranged pile of leaves, having a great time. He'd done all his work, and now it was time to play. So many good memories of those children.

Don:

After you sold the drive-in in 1983, you stayed in Millington for a few years?

Rosemary:

In Millington we lived across the street from the Whites, who asked us to go to Hawaii with them. How we did love it. Vivian was the most precise person, like my mother. We had such a good time doing all the things people do on their first trip to Hawaii. There is only one thing that I'd like to forget. Howard went down to the hot tub, where several young people were having a good time. Howard said, "Come on Rosemary, let's go down there."

I said, "I'm not going down there when all those young people are in the tub."

He went down to join them and started calling up to our balcony: "Rosemary, Rosemary."

I told Vivian White, "I'll give you five dollars to be Rosemary." Down she went and slid into the tub beside him. I'm sure he didn't know what was happening.

Our years in Millington had been good for us, because we had friends who were bankers, doctors, and politicians. Howard's favorite tennis partner was a state senator.

When we returned from Hawaii, we bought the Parkway House condo, where I've lived in for 17 years. You have visited almost every month since we recognized that Dad's memory was dying. He had Alzheimer disease, and I had denial. A good combination, wasn't it?

We had 10 years here together. In the six years since then, I've learned what being alone is like. I was alone for 20 years at the beginning of my life, and I'm going to have to take what comes now. But it has been a wonderful life, a wonderful experience. You can turn your hard luck into good luck. We have been as optimistically happy as anyone could ever be.

Interview 3: 1911–1999
Memories of Howard

Don:

This will be the third in a series of 2005 interviews with Rosemary Nicholson, Mama Nick, Mom. We'll talk about her memories of Howard Nicholson, born November 3, 1911 and died October 19, 1999. Where shall we begin?

Rosemary:

I met Howard when I was 14 and had finished the 10th grade. He was 18 and had graduated from high school. He had not only been an All-State quarterback and a newspaper celebrity, but also a basketball player on Classen's second place team at the national championships.

Don:

How did he arrive at the position of quarterback when his brother, four years older than Howard, had been an All-State center on the same team?

Rosemary:

He had practiced his head off. And Gaga, his mother—Mrs. Nicholson—trotted over to the practice field and told the coach that, although his brother had been a center, Howard should be a quarterback. Rather than have Gaga on his back for three years, the coach put him quarterback, and sure enough, he became All-State.

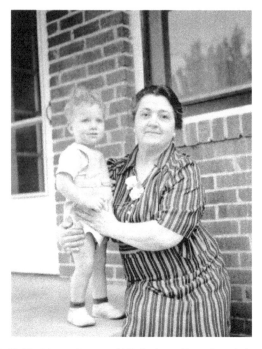

Fig. 23. 1943. Marie Prevratil Nicholson (Gaga) and the author.

His mother always loved football because both her boys had been high school stars. When I was on the team (being courted) and we went to a football game together, Mrs. Nicholson, five feet tall and round as a pumpkin, would get out of the car running so she wouldn't miss the kickoff. She was a very little woman and heavyset. Her mother was Prevratil from the Czech Republic.

Howard had graduated from high school the summer that I met him. We had that lovely summer together, and

I thought it would be for the rest of our lives. But the following year, I had to go to my grandparent's home in Bartlesville to live. Howard went to the University of Oklahoma (OU), having saved enough money after working as a delivery boy.

At OU he joined Phi Gamma Delta fraternity, working in the kitchen to earn his board. He enjoyed that one year as a fraternity member and proudly regarded himself a Fiji for the rest of his life. When I returned from Bartlesville, our courtship picked up again. We usually rode in Jack Fleming's little yellow car, a Ford Valencia. Howard and I sat in the rumble seat. We were living then in Oklahoma City but married in Tulsa.

Don:

Why did you marry in Tulsa?

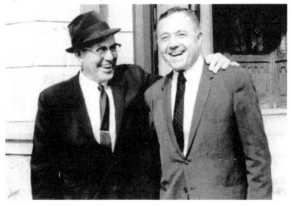

Fig. 24. 1952. Jack Fleming and Howard.

Rosemary:

All my years I've told people that it was because it our former pastor was now in Tulsa. But it really was because when I called our new preacher in Oklahoma City and told him the date we wanted to get married, he said he already had tickets to a football game for that day! How could a football game be more important than our wedding?

Don:

Tell us about the picture of you and Dad at the altar in Tulsa.

Rosemary:

Fifty years after the wedding, we visited Robert at his new home in Tulsa. We went to the chapel where we were married and posed for a photograph in front of the altar. When we returned home and developed the photograph, I was stunned to see my arms in the same position, my hands in the same position, and my feet in the same position as in our wedding photo. I guess we hadn't improved a bit over the past 50 years!

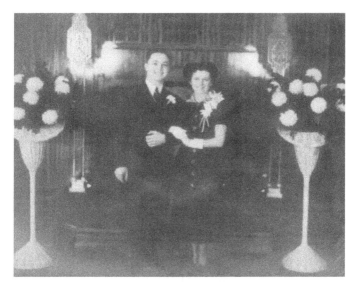

Fig. 25. Tulsa November 22, 1936.

Don:

Dad went to work for Paramount in 1932, during the Great Depression.

Rosemary:

Yes. He stood in a long line all day outside the Paramount branch office in Oklahoma City to be interviewed. At night the men in line agreed that each could go home, rinse off, put on a cleaner shirt, eat a bite, and return to the same place in line. Howard thought that by the time he got into the building, it would be his turn for the interview. Instead, the line inside stretched up to the second floor and out of sight! When they called him late that night to say he had the job, he asked, "Well, what will I wear?" He had told them everything about himself but didn't have any idea what job he was applying for.

He went first to the ad-sales department, which sells the big one-sheets that that advertise current and coming attractions in display cases outside the theater. Howard was then promoted to the shipping department, where they ship the film that theaters have rented. After that, he was promoted to salesman and traveled on a circuit to theaters around the state to "sell" pictures. This was actually a rental arrangement between Paramount's sales and distribution division and theaters based either on a flat fee for a stated duration, or, for new movies, a percentage of the theater's gross ticket sales. The flat fee at that time was small, probably $15 or $20, including shipping.

Don:

What was his starting salary?

Rosemary:

I am pretty sure it was $17.50 a week. He was able to ask me to marry him when he was promoted to traveling salesman—salary $35 a week. Reimbursement for his travel expenses by the company (expense account) added to the weekly salary. When he tried to turn in his expense account to the penny for what he had spent, the two other salesmen straightened him out: "Don't do that. They don't even check your expense account if it's under a hundred dollars." Howard padded along with the others.

As a wedding gift, we had received a ledger, which I used for years to record every penny of personal income and expenses.

Don:

How did you spend your weekends during the Dallas years?

Rosemary:

We had many memorable reunions in Dallas. Our Oklahoma friends always stayed with us for the OU–Texas football game in the Cotton Bowl. One weekend we sent both children to a sitter's house. We had guest beds in every room downstairs and up. I had put signs on the toilet seats. Those that were raised said "little boys' room." The seats that were down said "little girls' room." I'd walk into the dining room and find a man shaving in the buffet mirror. There were friends we invited and a few who tagged along with the crowd. What a lively memory!

Interview 4: 1985–2005
Odds and Ends

Don:

> This is the fourth interview with Rosemary Nicholson, Mama Nick, Mom. Is there anything else you'd like to say about the Dallas years before we move on to Memphis?

Rosemary:

> Howard took an evening business law course at SMU while he was with Paramount. He thought that many of his business interests required more legal background. For example, he invested in two commercial lots in Dallas, when the Trinity Industrial District was first developed in the 1950s. He bought them in a new area of empty land being developed for warehouses. You didn't even get to pick your lot. You picked the area, signed the contract, and the developer assigned the specific lots. There was only one tree on the whole place. Howard said, "If that tree is on my lot, I'll tie a cow to it." Sure enough, the tree was on his lot.

> One of the things he did when he was buying those two buildings at separate times, a year or two apart, was to ask my mother if she wanted a $5,000 share of one. He could afford it himself, but he wanted to give her the option. She said, "Indeed I do." And they partnered on that one. When he sold them in the 1970s and 1980s, we

were able to give Janet and Robert each $7,000 when they bought their first house.

The Variety Club was the nucleus of our friendship family in Dallas. I remember one night we stayed all night because they were trying to teach us how to do the "one, two, three kick" dance. It took all night, but we mastered it properly. We had lots of fun there.

Don:

In 1951 Howard was promoted from sales manager in Dallas to branch manager in Memphis.

Rosemary:

I had to stay behind as usual to sell the house. I came to Memphis for a weekend and put an ad in the paper to rent a house. Someone called at midnight the first night we were here, in bed at the Chisca Hotel, and told us we had won a car. Disappointed, I said, "Oh, I thought you were calling about a rental house." They never let me forget that.

Don:

I've heard many times that you won the car at the Variety Club the first week he was here, and the first Sunday you went to church, he gave 10 percent of the value of that car to the church.

Rosemary:

> We visited Trinity Church that Sunday. He started writing a check to Trinity. I wasn't even considering joining there. "Don't you want to wait until you know which church you're going to?"
>
> He said, "No. If I wait, I'll get stingy."

Don:

> A few years after you had moved to Memphis, you found a house that you really loved, 1819 Forrest Avenue. Would you tell me about that?

Rosemary:

> You talked about the things Howard did in Dallas that showed his good business sense. I'll give you a Memphis example. Dad looked at the contract and told the seller's attorney, "You didn't include the vacant lot." Sure enough, the contract did not include the proper dimensions of the property. They had to redraw the contract and give us the lot on the east side of the house. I would never in the world have known it was missing. The omission was intentional, I'm sure.
>
> Robert was born in February that year, and Howard was elected Chief Barker (president) of the Memphis Variety Club. This charitable group had already acquired land on Manassas Street and started constructing a hospital for children with rheumatic heart disease. He got it

completed during his term of office and won the international prize for the Variety Club Best Charity, which that year was presented to us in Toronto. We were popping with pride! [The hospital later became part of St. Jude Children's Research Hospital.]

Don:

Tell me about the Forrest house and Dad's work on it.

Rosemary:

The interior had woodwork, moldings, windows, and frames covered with thick layers of dark oil because the heating system had been a coal furnace. Howard started cleaning the woodwork and it looked better, but not a lot. He then stripped it all—probably what he should have done in the first place. The result was a beautiful gum woodwork throughout the house.

Don:

I was away at Stanford at the time. It must have taken months of hard weekend labor.

Rosemary:

Yes.

Don:

The Memphis years ended in 1963, when Dad was transferred as branch manager to Pittsburgh. Can you tell us about life in Pittsburgh?

Rosemary:

It was a disappointment to move, because we were having such a good time in Memphis. We rented a house in Mount Lebanon from the people who lived next door. They had to take the railing off of the staircase to get Janet's piano in!

The only defect, invisible to Tennesseans renting the house in summer, was the long driveway that swooped down behind the house. A coronary shoveling exercise in winter. After he had gotten up each morning, adjusted earmuffs and hat, donned gloves, mopped up and swept up and chopped up enough ice and snow to get his car out, Howard said, "I'll bet they were waiting for some damned southerner to come up here and rent this house!"

Don:

Tell us what it was like having Robert as the only child in the house.

Rosemary:

Everyone was friendly to Robert and accepting in school. In wintertime, they froze the tennis courts, and Howard and Robert ice skated on the surface. It was lighted at night, and a teacher was on duty. They had a wonderful place to skate. Howard grew up in Iowa and was still a super-skater!

Don:

That was the peak of his career with Paramount.

Rosemary:

His final year he made $15,000. That was the most he made in the whole 30 years he had been on their payroll. What has permitted us to live to a ripe old age is that he bought the drive-in theater in Millington.

Don:

You spent a couple of years in Millington after he retired. He had some other pastimes, didn't he?

Rosemary:

He loved to play tennis. At his age, that should be a joke, but it wasn't to him. It was a very serious game, even after surgery to replace both hips. A friend Don's age, Bobby Bostick, told me: "I never saw a man want to win as bad as Howard. I tried to tell him, 'Don't chase a ball that's going out of bounds, because you're going to miss the next two.' But he continued trying to hit every ball."

Don:

When he sold the drive-in, in 1983, he was offered less money by the leading theater chain in the area than he thought it was worth. To try to convince him, Malco sent executives, their real estate group, and a couple of drive-in owners in the area who had sold to Malco. Since there were no other markets, Dad created his own—a very attractive sign that he put in front of the theater with all of the information, price, terms, payments, everything. He sold it himself within a year for a much better price than the bargain that Malco had been seeking.

Rosemary:

The buyer of the property put several different businesses on the land. It now features a Walmart Superstore on one side, an Ace Hardware on the other, with ample parking for both, plus a discount store that I can't remember. The projection booth and concession stand are still intact and deserve a Tennessee State Historical Marker! We were through with our years and tears of trying to maintain and improve the drive-in.

Don:

Dad's retirement years were from 1983 to 1999. His Alzheimer disease took the last 10 years of his life. Can you tell us what he was like in his retirement years prior to that disease?

Rosemary:

We bought this condo, where I still live. When we first walked into the place, it seemed like we had just walked into a candy store. Completely furnished and decorated exquisitely by a gay couple who had both died from AIDS. It had been vacant for a year, and we would've taken it in a minute. Janet and two of her friends had an estate sale at our Millington house and wouldn't let either of us come to help or watch. Janet knew that I would have said, "You're not going to sell that for five dollars, are you?"

After we moved here in April, 1984, Howard had five good years. We returned to Trinity Methodist Church and were near our Forrest house, so the location was comfortable. Dad was even elected chairman of the condo board.

Near the end it was harder to take care of him. Once I slept on the floor in the living room with him because he had fallen and I couldn't get him up. I didn't want him to be frightened if he awakened, so I just got my pillow and blanket, cuddled down beside him, and we had a fine time. I don't think he ever knew that he would've been in danger without me, because I was just supposed to be there.

Don:

"Sacrifice" was not part of your vocabulary. When you spent those last years of his life here with him in this condominium, instead of putting him in a nursing home, it was not a sacrifice for you. That was simply part of your love, part of your life, and a natural part of what life had in store for you.

Rosemary:

Yes.

Don:

This ends my last interview session with Mom. I'm sorry I didn't know how to do the recordings and transcriptions while Dad was alive. Memories alone don't do him justice. From all of us, Mom, thank you for this time, your patience, humor, wisdom, and your talent as a performer.

PART 3:

RETIREMENT YEARS

Chapter 15

Hurricane Recoveries

Hurricane Andrew, 1992

Our first indication that we might be in for trouble came Sunday evening, August 23, 1992. To increase his hand–eye coordination and manual dexterity, Keith's counselor had recommended he do some exercises with nuts, bolts, and holes drilled in plywood boards. I thought that making the boards myself might enhance my own handyman ability and self-esteem, so we headed together to Home Depot after dinner. The place was mobbed. Magda and Keith were borne away by a sea of frantic customers. While I was squeezing my way to the nuts and bolts aisle, a lady with a sheet of plywood slammed into me.

"Sorry," she said. "I was in a hurry to get out of here before the crowd gets any bigger!"

"What's the matter?" I asked.

"Hurricane," she called as she shouldered her way to the cashier.

I then began to pay more attention to comments around me and less to plans in my head. A Category 5 hurricane was headed our way, scheduled to arrive in a few hours. I found Keith and Magda, and we returned home.

Our lack of hurricane preparation gave us more time to plan sleeping arrangements. Magda's sister, Eva, was alone in her house with her son, Trevor, and they decided that they would be safer with us. That put Magda, Kata, and Eva in the master bedroom. Jim Tiedeman, a visiting ophthalmologist from Duke, and I put our mattresses in the hallway. Keith, Dax, and Trevor stayed in the children's bedroom.

Once sleeping arrangements were settled, Eva lit a cigarette. It was midnight, and wind was beginning to howl. I calmly told Eva to throw the cigarette out the front door into the gathering storm, or I would do the same to her. She thought a moment, listened to the wind, and threw the cigarette out the front door.

Jim and I parked the cars to shelter as best we could the sliding glass doors/walls, then stuffed towels under the sliding doors. So ended our preparation for Hurricane Andrew.

We lived on the northern boundary of Andrew's Category 5 winds, 175mph at landfall. Our home was on an acre surrounded by mature pine and oak trees, whose trunks were silhouetted at 30- to 45-degree angles from the vertical during the night by periodic bursts of white light. They were bent but generally not broken by the fierce wind. Periodically a deafening explosion and thud would signal a splitting trunk and falling tree. Andrew was a fast-traveling storm that roared through like a runaway train, leaving behind little rain. A few crabs landed on our street, blown two miles from Biscayne Bay. There was no significant tidal surge or flooding. At dawn the wind died, and we went outside to check the damage. We had no hurricane shutters or hurricane impact widows. Nevertheless, our beautiful wood-paneled glass sliding doors on two sides of the living-family room were intact. Walls and windows were intact. A few roof tiles were missing and the pool screen was blown out, but that was all. The surrounding grove of pines and oaks had absorbed the force of the wind and blocked projectiles. The trees were our protective barrier.

Our worst experience was living through the last two months of Miami summer without electricity. Buying ice took hours of wheeling a cooler by hand along the street. There was no gasoline available because filling stations had no generators. No electricity, no gas. Magda spent a half day lugging home a block of ice, with which she had hoped to cool her face and fix a glass of ice water. I put a package of chicken into the ice and consequently bloodied it. I turned on the propane barbecue to begin preparing dinner.

"Chicken," she screamed. "You want chicken?" She plucked the chicken from the bloody ice and threw it on the grill. "Well, here's your chicken," she shrieked, pushing fiery grill, propane tank, and chicken into the swimming pool.

The tank gurgled as it sank. To appreciate the full effect, you must understand that Magda pronounces it "shicken." As in, "Let's go chopping for shicken at the market."

Because Miami supplies were still exhausted, during one of my monthly Memphis visits I bought a chain saw. In mid-September I bought a Honda gasoline generator from the back of a truck that had hauled a load of them from central Florida. A few stations were now selling gas if you had cash and patience. During our last six weeks we had the luxuries of a box fan and refrigerator supplied with power from our own generator.

When the Georgia Power crew drove to our house on mid-October to reconnect our electricity, the whole family paraded out to greet them, cheering "Go D-A-W-G-S" at the top of our lungs.

Hurricane Dennis, 2005

In 1997 I bought three vacant lots and a one-story CBS house, on Carrabelle Beach, FL. The house was isolated on a pristine white beach with sand so fine that it squeaked beneath our feet when we walked. We saw horseshoe crabs mating and sea turtles nesting in their seasons. Most interesting of all were our new, small-town friends.

I'll tell about only one, Herbert Mock. Born into a big family of Carrabelle Mocks, Herbert had weathered the gulf for 70 years. He adopted me as a friend and introduced me to Franklin County culture.

"When I was a boy, I went to the beach near your house to hunt turtle eggs," he explained. "I used a straightened coat hanger, walked along where I thought they was nests, and stuck my coat hanger into the sand. When it went through, I knew I'd found the nest. I dug up the eggs and took 'em to Mom. She used 'em to make the best angel food cake ever." I'd like to take his mother's turtle-egg angel food cake recipe to our next Gulf Conservationist meeting.

He also described the madness of the annual Father–Son Fishing Tournament in Carrabelle. "They's so many cars, so many people. You'd think you was in ..." He wrinkled his brow and repeated, "You'd think you was in ... Tallahassee!" That was the boundary of Herbert's world.

The key to Carrabelle's future economic development? Herbert agreed with Carrabelle's long-time mayor, Curley Messer. "We should convince someone to build a McDonald's in Carrabelle. Would your son Keith [age 16] do it?" Unfortunately, Herbert died from Covid-19 in 2020, before there was a Carrabelle McDonald's.

Carrabelle Beach was our escape, a 12-hour drive from Miami, with a Walmart in Chiefland for Magda's shopping break and Bett's Big T Restaurant for lunch. Kata moved to

Tampa after a few years, so a night with her, Brenan, and Sara was an extra joy at the halfway point.

In 2005 Hurricane Dennis flooded the house with a four-foot tidal surge. We learned about Dennis a bit late, while we were in Ashville, NC, celebrating Magda's birthday. I had thought the storm would hit too far west to cause damage to our beach house, but *USA Today* had an article about the hurricane flooding Ouzt's Too Oyster Bar on the Wakulla River, 45 miles east of Carrabelle Beach. I realized instantly that our house had been in the flood zone, but it took four days for me to drive Magda home to Coral Gables, and an additional day for me to drive to Carrabelle. I arrived on the eleventh day after the hurricane.

The house was intact, but three feet of green muck and black mold covered the floor and lower walls. I had no experience in flood recovery, but a dear neighbor, Henry Reed, had survived several hurricanes with flooding. He was an experienced, knowledgeable, and skilled friend. The morning after I arrived, he pulled a wet-vac and a gasoline-powered pressure cleaner down the street to my house and showed me how to use them to get rid of the muck. After I had removed damp drywall, sprayed fungicide to kill mold, and shocked myself with a water-soaked 120-volt electrical outlet, I hired Henry as handyman, carpenter, and electrician. He had already suffered two recurrences of Vietnam Agent Orange-induced lymphoma, but he worked long and hard through summer heat to help me. My sister Janet and her husband Larry drove from Memphis in September to finish drywall replacement with me. We bought a how-to-replace-drywall book at Ace Hardware. Thirteen years later the same book floated to the surface of Hurricane Michael's flood in the garage.

After Hurricane Dennis, I installed hurricane shutters and shatter-proof windows, elevated the air conditioner on a six-foot high platform, replaced the water heater with a tank-less model mounted six feet above floor level in the garage, and installed doors that opened to the outside to discourage flood water from entering the house. These improvements might have been sufficient for hurricanes past, but they were no match for Michael.

Hurricane Michael, 2018

In October 2018 from Miami, I monitored the course of Hurricane Michael as it moved north through the Gulf of Mexico and headed directly for our part of the Florida panhandle. Michael made landfall as a Category 5 hurricane October 18 at Mexico Beach, 50 miles west of Carrabelle. The side of the storm east of the eye was the strong side, the "dirty" side, the side that hit our house. Before I left Miami, I called Angie Printiss, an excellent Carrabelle carpenter who had helped me with some previous improvements. I hired her to meet me on the third morning after Michael hit. Luckily, electricity had been restored the night before. The front of the house looked untouched as I approached from the street. On the beach side an eight-foot tidal surge had lifted the storm awnings out of the track and shattered hurricane windows and sliding glass doors.

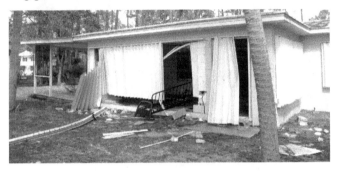

Fig. 26. South side of beach house three days after the eight-foot Hurricane Michael tidal surge.

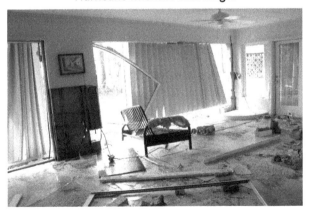

Fig. 27. Interior view of battered hurricane shutters and broken shatter-proof windows and sliding glass doors.

The surge had floated refrigerator, TV, sofas, chairs, and dining table across the living room, dining area, and kitchen, and smashed them against the intact north wall of the kitchen, depositing the jumbled, broken pile of furniture on a thick layer of thick "shatter-proof" shards.

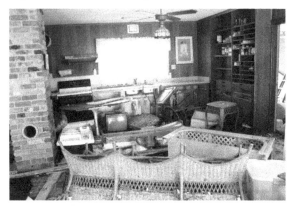

Fig. 28. Furniture and appliances smashed into broken kitchen cabinets by the surge.

The wooden deck outside the family room had floated upward, tethered only at the two sides, anchored to bedroom and sunroom walls. The southwest, untethered corner of the deck, pushed the metal roof upward, bending it. The central air conditioner, mounted on a six-foot-high deck of eight-inch timber pilings, and the duct system were flooded by seawater. On the first day I drove three miles to the FEMA center and arranged for a volunteer to help me the following morning. Bright and sort of early, Charlie Boyer, owner and publisher of *Jazz & Blues Florida* arrived with muscle and ingenuity to scrape shattered glass, muck, and debris from the floor with a snow shovel I had kept from my Boston days. Charlie then helped us tote the doorless broken refrigerator to the swale and lay it on its back to serve as a receptacle for broken glass and debris. He was with us for a full week. Between stints publishing a monthly compendium of blues and jazz events throughout Florida, Boyer drives to volunteer in disaster areas all over the country. What a guy!

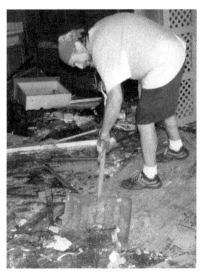

Fig. 29. Charlie Boyer wielding a snow shovel.

Now I want to tell you about "Wonder Woman", who used true superpowers to restore the structural integrity of this battered beach house. Angie Printiss, housewife and mother of a college freshman daughter, is a world-class carpenter. On her own, she removed loosened concrete blocks and shattered glass doors and windows, then designed and built frames to support sheets of half-inch plywood to shield the interior of the house. Angie also replaced sheet rock and kitchen cabinets.

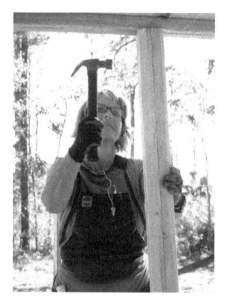

Fig. 30. Angie Prentiss, "Wonder Woman".

After eleven days she had created a weatherproof cabin that would permit me to continue the next two years of observing, haggling with, and overpaying a purgatory series of local contractors with varying degrees of dependability, honesty, and skill–with laborers to match.

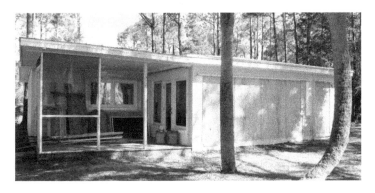

Fig. 31. After 11 days of "Wonder Woman".

My main roles in the project were accountant, paymaster, and garbageman.

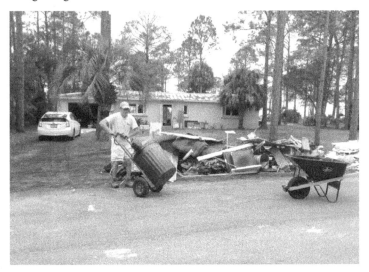

Fig. 32. My main role.

Once again, I incorporated lessons learned into my hurricane repair plans. I replaced the central air conditioner with two mini-split units positioned on east and west exterior walls eight feet above the ground, or 11 feet above sea level. I anchored the wooden deck/screened porch to a 600-pound block of concrete buried in the sand. I reduced the size of replacement hurricane-proof windows on the beach side of the house to reduce the pressure that could be exerted by a tidal surge that rises to window level. Hurricane shutters are a liability in a tidal surge, so I did not replace the shutters that lifted out of their tracks. After the repairs were complete I sold the house and lots. I hoped to retire from my hurricane repair career, but still living in Florida makes that unlikely.

Chapter 16

Fidel's Shadow in Cuban Miami

For 50 years I have lived among relatives, friends, neighbors, colleagues, patients, and workers whose lives were torn apart by the 1959 Cuban Revolution. In no other U.S. city would I have learned first-hand the strength, courage, resilience, resourcefulness, and perseverance that I have encountered innumerable times among these victims. With the help of my own fluent Spanish and my extrovert Cuban wife, I have been able to catch many ripples that would have otherwise passed an Oklahoma gringo unnoticed. Many of our mundane daily tasks are intertwined with Fidel.

One example was an emergency plumbing repair interrupted by a meeting to plot a counter-revolution.

Carlos Valdez (not his real name) was a 17-year-old engineering student in Havana at the time of the revolution. He fought against Castro's rebels, was captured, tortured, and imprisoned for 21 years. At age 38 he came to Miami and worked as an apprentice plumber, earning his license after 10 years. After 10 more years of hard work and frugal living, he had saved enough money to start his own company.

One Friday night in 1990 we were awakened by a roar of gushing water under our house. We called Carlos's emergency number, and one of his employees came to turn off our water. The main water pipe under our house had burst.

The next day his crew—minus Carlos—arrived. After exploring the damage to pipes under the house, two of the men argued about which method to use for repair.

"Why don't you call Carlos?" I asked.

"Because he's in Nicaragua this week," replied one. "Plotting a counter-revolution in Cuba," added the other.

Rather than rely on either of the two arguing assistants for definitive repair, we decided to await Carlos's return. Only in Miami might one encounter a delay in an emergency plumbing repair because the boss was in Nicaragua planning an invasion of Cuba.

Chapter 17

Travels with Magda

To the Border

We have visited most of the world, between international congresses during my working years and retirement. The experiences have provided material for hundreds of PowerPoint presentations to children and grandchildren, with active participation by the whole family on a good day. My most memorable trip with Magda, though, was right here in Miami to the doorstep of death. In 1987, two years after Keith's birth, Magda was two months pregnant. We thought all was well, with normal initial OB visits. She was working as my secretary. One afternoon, returning from South Miami, she started bleeding heavily. She continued driving 10 miles to the entrance of Bascom Palmer, saturating the gray cloth seat of the Honda with blood and fainting in shock. Attendants at the front door immediately called an ambulance, and she was taken across the street to the Jackson Memorial Hospital emergency room. She stabilized after several units of blood.

The surgeon said that the embryo had been implanted on the cervix, instead of inside the uterus, and doctors had not been able to stop the bleeding after loss of the embryo. An emergency hysterectomy was the only way to save her life.

As they wheeled the gurney to the OR, she was fading in and out of consciousness. She opened her eyes long enough to say, "Take care of Dax and Kata."

"Of course," I replied as the door to surgery closed behind her. At that moment I was certain that the boatman would not yet take her across. When she awoke in the recovery room, she called to ask that I bring her cosmetics kit.

Panama and Telluride: August, 1987

By late June 1987 the news from Panama had darkened. Street fighting and demonstrations against Manuel Noriega, dictator of Panama, grew more violent. The military began shooting demonstrators with shotguns loaded with birdshot, generally causing only superficial wounds to skin struck by pellets. When birdshot hits the eyeball, however, it can penetrate the sclera and damage delicate structures inside—lens, retina, optic nerve—leaving the eye filled with blood and birdshot remnants. Emergency management of these injuries required a relatively recent type of surgery, pars plana vitrectomy, developed and first used at Bascom Palmer in 1970. The procedure was not available to ophthalmologists in Panama when these injuries began to be inflicted, and very few of the victims had resources to travel to the United States for care. Many eyes remained permanently blind.

I contacted Benjamin F. Boyd, M.D. (1925–2018), a friend and respected leader of Panamanian and international ophthalmology to ask if I might help. We decided that I should bring a team to Panama, using my connections at Bascom Palmer, and ask Alcon to sponsor a medical mission to provide vitrectomy equipment, medical supplies, and technical personnel. In Panama, Ben would facilitate connections with government and medical officials to secure the necessary permits.

My one-month Colorado family vacation was to begin the first of August. Telluride, then a laid-back ski resort, was new territory for our whole family, and we were anxious to explore. I had rented a three-bedroom house on W. Colorado Avenue well in advance of the August dates. By late July Ben said he was getting close to an agreement with the government and the ophthalmological society.

I decided to go ahead with our family vacation, crossing my fingers and hoping that Latin time would remain lazy.

Wandering downtown the morning after we arrived, we found an advertisement for a Grateful Dead concert in Town Park August 15 and 16. I called Darrell in Key Biscayne, told him, and he flew to Telluride to join the group. We bought tickets for Darrell, Dax, and Kata. Keith, age four, stayed with Magda and me in the house. Before The Grateful Dead concert, we had taken a rafting trip down the Green River rapids, visited Capitol Reef and Canyonlands National Parks, and stopped in Durango.

In Panama, street violence and ocular pellet injuries had increased. By mid-August the medical mission had been approved. Ben said I should prepare to leave by August 20. I left Telluride August 18 to drive the rental car to Miami for my flight. This left Magda alone with three children and only her feet for transportation.

At a Holiday Inn near Dallas that night, my secretary called and said the mission had been canceled by the Panamanian Health Council. Diplomatic entanglements won the day. I didn't learn the details until a year later in a publication by Physicians for Human Rights.

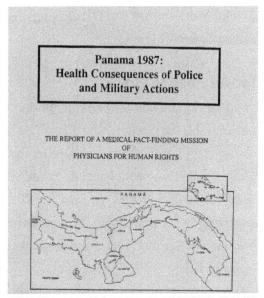

We queried Dr. Sanchez about the ocular bird shot wounds
which had been reported by the Eye Association, and asked him to
comment about Dr. Donald Nicholson of the Bascolm Palmer Eye
Institute of Miami who had been invited to Panama by the
Panamanian Eye Association to help care for these patients. Dr.
Sanchez says that this request was presented to the Panamanian
Health Council; the Council decided that Dr. Nicholson could
come only as a consultant but could not directly participate in
patient care because he was not licensed to practise medicine in
Panama. Dr. Sanchez mentioned that Dr. Michael DeBakey was not
permitted to operate on the Shah of Iran in Panama for similar
reasons.

Fig. 33. Panama 1987. Physicians for Human Rights. I was barred
from treating birdshot ocular wounds in Panama for the same
reason that Dr. Michael DeBakey of Houston had been barred
from operating on the Shah of Iran.

In October, 1989, President George H. W. Bush ordered
U.S. military forces to invade Panama. Noriega was captured

January 3, 1990. Neither I nor Dr. DeBakey was responsible for those events, as far as I know.

Turkey Hot-Air Balloon Crash

We spent two weeks touring all parts of Turkey and had dozens of memorable experiences, but I'll tell only one. In Cappadocia we stayed in Uçhisar, a village in the heart of the soft volcanic tuff stone area, where deep and steep-sided streams created tower-like shapes. In the early Bronze Age, man began carving living quarters in the soft stone. In subsequent centuries they created rock-cut houses, monasteries, and underground cities.

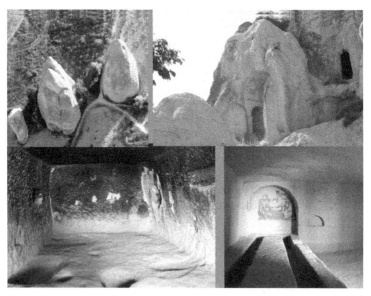

Fig. 33. Cappadocia.

One morning we reserved a hot-air balloon ride to see the mystical terrain from above. We had paid in advance. On the day of the flight, one of our companions canceled, giving no reason. The rest of us boarded our vans for the takeoff area. We watched the balloon inflate, the captain take command, and the gondola stabilized for the six passengers to board.

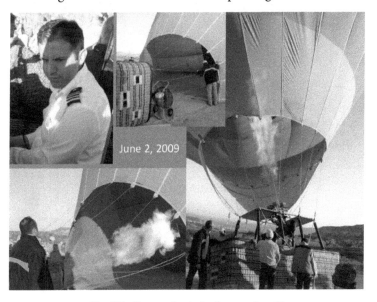

June 2, 2009

Fig. 35. Cappadocia balloon takeoff.

The view was mesmerizing. A dozen colorful balloons in crystal clear sky, ancient communities carved into towering rock towers in the valleys below, stone castles and churches passing in a dream.

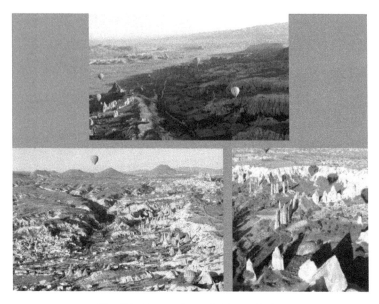

Fig. 36. Cappadocia balloon flight.

Finally, the captain reduced the flame, air cooled, and we descended to earth. Vans careened over desert floor to our landing spot, we climbed from the gondola, raised a champagne toast, and posed for a photograph.

When we returned to the hotel, our canceling friend greeted us. "How was the day? Tell me about the flight. Do you have pictures?" That evening over Uçhisar wine, he told us the story.

The day before our flight he learned that a hot air balloon in our area had descended rapidly and crashed into another below, sending both balloons crumbling to the ground. Dr. Kevin Beurle, a British space scientist, was killed and several others injured, one critically.

Our companion canceled his reservation and had kept it to himself. He didn't want to spoil the trip for the rest of us. We had enjoyed our day, unfettered by fear. A psychiatrist couldn't have done a better job.

Napa Earthquake: August 24, 2014

Magda and I were sound asleep in our room at the Fairmont Sonoma Mission Inn at three-thirty in the morning, when our king-size bed suddenly began to shake violently and bang against the wall. I knew from my years at Stanford that this was an earthquake, stronger than any I had felt before. I immediately grabbed Magda's shoulders and rolled us off the bed, onto the floor next to the wall, covering her with my body.

"What are you doing?" she shouted.

"Earthquake!"

"No, it's not. The air conditioner is broken." Apparently, earthquakes are not common in Cuba.

The Napa 6.0 magnitude earthquake of 2014 was the strongest in the area since the Loma Prieta earthquake in 1989. We were scheduled to start our Johns Hopkins travel group tour of the Napa Valley wine country that same morning. We followed orders, exited our room, and waited outside with other hotel guests and employees for two hours, until state building inspectors verified that there was no structural damage to the hotel. At noon we drove the 30 miles from Sonoma to Napa and found damage from the earthquake was more severe.

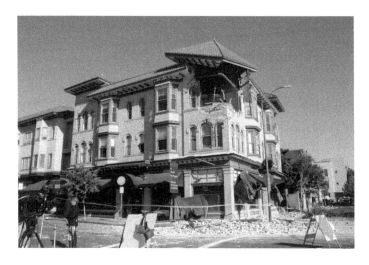

Fig. 37. Ground Zero in downtown Napa for earthquake photographers, telecasts, and interviews.

Mississippi Delta Blues

Clarksdale MS. The Crossroads, where sin (blues) and salvation (gospel) split.

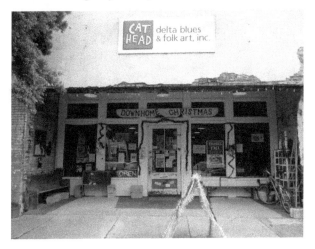

Fig. 38. Clarksdale, MS. Cat Head Delta Blues & Folk Art.

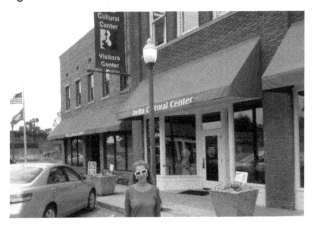

Fig. 39. Delta Cultural Center, Helena AR. Best blues museum in the Delta.

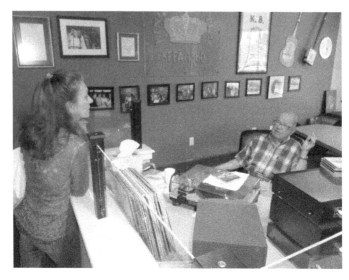

Fig. 40. Helena AR Delta Cultural Center. "Sunshine" Sonny Paine (1925–2018), KFFA blues radio host from 1951 until his death.

The Yazoo-Mississippi delta, where the blues were born, is a musical, historical, visual experience that invites you to explore the unique delta culture. Its history includes a Yellow Dog railroad story in Tutwiler, a songwriter for blackface Alabama minstrel shows turned bandleader and icon (W.C. Handy), a Founding Father with at least three reputed burial sites (Robert Johnson), a searing image of American racial cruelty and injustice in Money (Emmet Till), and a mother's courage (Mamie Till-Mobley).

Mamie Till-Mobley and Mass School Shootings

With every school shooting Mamie Till-Mobley comes to mind. She had her brutally murdered son, Emmett Till, brought from the Tutwiler MS Funeral Home to Chicago in a sealed coffin. There, courage and perspective compelled her to insist on an open coffin funeral to confront the world with the savagery of his fatal assault—his pistol-whipped, unrecognizable face, an eye ripped from the socket, a bullet hole in his head. *Jet Magazine* was equally courageous in publishing photographs that showed Emmet's viciously destroyed face to the world.

With her act of defiance, Mamie Till-Mobley contributed a cornerstone of the Civil Rights movement. What would she advise relatives of murdered children and teachers to do today after a mass school shooting?

No longer do we need newspaper chains or large news organizations to put a stamp of approval on what is appropriate for public view. Social media, perhaps with techie help, will spread the images worldwide in seconds. By dealing with the pain and grief of an open casket decision, parents and other relatives can by themselves awaken voters, politicians, and businesses to defend against this cruel, senseless tragedy.

There is no better place to begin your delta visit than Clarksdale, MS. We also loved Helena AR, across the Mississippi, but, sadly, "Sunshine" Sonny Paine died a few years ago.

Favorite Blues Joint in Clarksdale

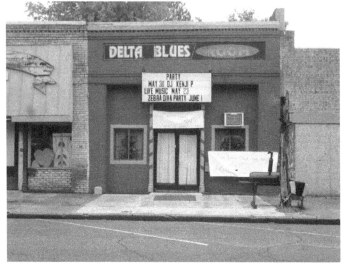

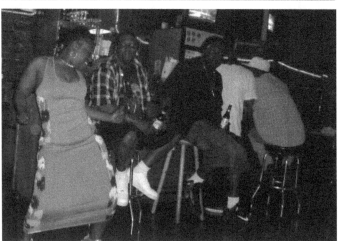

Fig. 41. Clarksdale Delta Blues Room.

Chapter 18

Farewell to Medicine

I left the University of Miami in 1994 and went into private practice in Coral Gables for two years. For several years, I had taken courses in practice management, the business side of medical practice. Maybe that could be an area in which I might continue a medial career after I had passed my peak surgical ability.

A successful Miami ophthalmologist wanted to sell his practice and retire. He had a corporate buyer, but he needed someone to continue clinical and surgical practice plus manage his office, which included three ophthalmologists, one optometrist, a surgical center, nurses, technicians, and administrative staff. It looked like a good fit.

The practice side was challenging, rewarding, and enjoyable, as it had been at the university. One of my referred patients had won the Nobel Peace Prize.

The administrative side was a good learning experience, always a source of enjoyment. After two years, the group that had purchased our practice was absorbed by a larger group, and I was fired to cut costs.

One of my first free weekdays after being flushed into retirement, I made a long-postponed routine visit to my internist. The nurse led me to the scale. One hundred and ninety pounds! I had abandoned my health somewhere along the line. My career path was now clear. I had to transfer my obsessive–compulsive side from medicine to exercise.

Chapter 19

Marathon Man

Over a two-year period I gradually progressed from walking around the block to running 5K and 10K races. I added a marathon nine-month group training the next year and began to run half-marathons. First the ING Miami, then on two of my monthly Memphis visits, the St. Jude Half. Finally, my Sunday long run extended to 20 miles, from home in Coral Gables, through Coconut Grove, over the 80-foot-high Rickenbacker Causeway Bridge ("the Miami mountain") to Key Biscayne and back. That spring at age 66, I ran my first full marathon, the Nashville Country Music Marathon. Country music bands and singers were placed along the 26.2-mile course, about one group per mile.

It was an exhilarating celebration of the 40 years since I had completed my internal medicine internship at Vanderbilt University Hospital.

In 2008 I also finished Miami and Sarasota marathons. The latter was no longer held after that year. I hope I didn't break it.

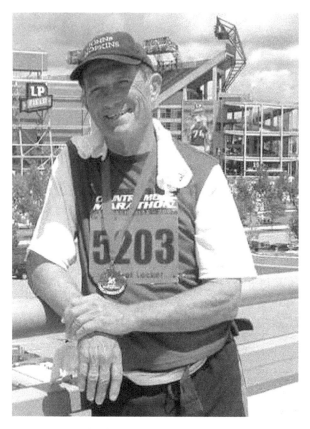

Fig. 42. Nashville 2007 Country Music Marathon.

Running became an integral part of enjoying life, both in Miami and when we traveled. Dawn in Paris from Place de la Concorde, through Trocadero, across the Seine, beneath Eiffel Tower, back across the river, and around the Louvre to Concorde, beating the morning traffic.

In Istanbul I ran from Europe to Asia and back. The Virginia Creeper Trail near Abington shows what can be built for the public from investment in abandoned railroad tracks.

At age 70 heart trouble and its treatment reduced my exercise tolerance and ended my long-distance running. I have since used a brisk three-mile walk each day, push-ups, barbells, and core exercises to stay in condition. I now weigh 158.

Chapter 20

Teaching

When I left the university in 1994, I was still using 35mm slides and Carousel projectors to teach classes. I then began to prepare digital presentations with PowerPoint to show grandchildren our travel adventures. We gathered around my PC on folding chairs, grandchildren on the first row, children on the second, telephones locked away. Interjections and questions from the front row drove the presentation. Laughter, conversation, and communication flowed—magical family experiences.

I returned to Bascom Palmer as a volunteer to teach medical students once a week for 10 years. With this experience my travel presentations improved, according to the grandchildren.

The Osher Lifelong Learning Institute at the University of Miami let me improve my teaching style even more. With internet and PowerPoint, I could now volunteer to teach the subject on the list I knew least about, thereby learning much more myself. During a one-year period, for example, I taught classes to the group on Rwanda, Darfur, Central Asia Republics, and the US–China trade balance. During the pandemic I also learned to teach via Zoom.

Chapter 21

Gardening

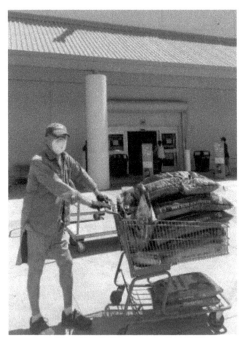

Fig. 43. Garden supplies for the 2020 Covid-19 lockdown.

I then entered the realm of true geezerdom—gardening. I respect your perfectly normal response to this topic—skip to the next chapter. Before you do, let me give you an example of the fun you can find in the field.

I learned to include audio and visual attachments in PowerPoint presentations.

When I presented a Zoom talk to the Tropical Rose Society on the "Nitty-Gritty of Rose Weeding and Mulching," I concluded with Florida Georgia Line's rendition of "Dirt." I told the audience that I could not use the Nitty-Gritty Dirt Band because their New Jersey origin doesn't let them inspire South Florida rose growers.

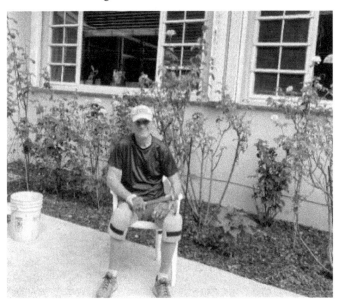

Fig. 44. 2022 Showtime: Tropical Rose Society "Nitty-Gritty Rose Weeding and Mulching" via Zoom.

Chapter 22

The COVID-19 Pandemic

About a year-and a-half into the Covid-19 pandemic, I realized that this was not our only pandemic. We had been isolated for so long that loneliness had begun to creep in and take over. Loneliness that laughed at Zoom Meeting cures.

Gardening helped some. It did not, of course, replace the lack of human contact. Roses blooming, gladiolas thriving, orchids surprising me with new blooms, the fragrance of white butterfly ginger—all brought solace. However, the few times I did interact with others, I found my verbal ability withering away. My words and sentences didn't come out right. I had to repeat myself. I couldn't understand others' speech as well as before. Denial was still my defense strategy for the cognitive disorder/dementia diagnoses five years before.

My writing ability held up pretty well. In 2020 I began writing a memoir for grandchildren, which was therapeutic and reassuring.

Another band-aid was my reading appetite. I always have several books on my reading table. They give me, among other things, vicarious human connection. Javier Zamora's *Solito*, Vivek Murthy's *Together*, and Michael Bulgakov's *The Master and Margarita* are three I hope you read someday.

In spite of these efforts, loneliness remained. When in-class instruction resumed at OLLI @ UM, I jumped at the chance to escape the Zoom cage. Pencil drawing and creative writing were the first two in-class courses I saw in the catalog. I picked the latter, and it worked. Within a few weeks, I had new friends, and my speech began to improve—not yet normal, but better.

After two semesters, I moved to Improv 101.

This course was a magic bullet. My recommendation for breaking out of the pandemic loneliness trap is an in-person Improv course. The problem, of course, is that Improv requires memory as much as imagination, in order to react instantly to the comments of fellow students. I retired from Improv after three six-week courses.

Chapter 23

OLLI (Osher Lifelong Learning Institute) at UM

Creative Writing 2022

Addiction

Four generations of addiction. Where should I begin? Grandfather, uncle, brother, sister, stepson ... me? I won't write about suicide generations because it's not part of our assignment. So, I'll start with me, the most recently diagnosed—in my ninth decade.

After reading Vivek Murthy's excellent book *Together*, I realized for the first time that I have had a lifelong addiction to academic achievement and recognition. Top reader in Miss Romine's kindergarten, straight A's, Honor Society, junior year Phi Beta Kappa at Stanford, AOA honor society in medical school, residency at Harvard and Hopkins, Professor of Ophthalmology, etc., etc., etc.

Murthy says, "doing gave [me] a false sense of control and stability. All the external markers kept telling [me] that I was a 'success,' even though I sensed the emotional hole in my life." I didn't recognize this until Rafael Cortez, a dear friend and colleague from Caracas gave me the book *Emotional Intelligence* by Daniel Goleman 20 years ago.

"Your I.Q. is tops; your E.Q. needs work," he said. An honest assessment from a kind friend.

Rewind Bar and Grille

Sam Bankman-Fried walks into a bar, Rewind, on Flatbush Avenue and sits on a barstool. The burley tattooed owner, Pat Sheehan, ambles over: "We've been expecting you."

"You knew I was coming?"

"Guilty of money laundering and securities fraud with both your parents on the Stanford Law School faculty? I knew you were coming."

"We've filed appeals," Bankman-Fried snaps.

"You didn't come here for legal counsel. You're here for a rewind."

"Where do I start?" Bankman-Fried's eyes dart around the bar.

"Right over there," Sheehan points to a door on the inside wall.

A stranger in a white jacket carrying a black leather bag hangs a sign on the door: Barber. Without a word, Bankman-Fried starts to follow him.

"Leave your laptop and phone on the bar," orders Sheehan.

An hour later, Bankman-Fried emerges, head bald as ivory. Behind him the barber carries a waste basket filled with Bankman-Fried's never washed or combed black, curly locks.

"Why did he shave my eyebrows?" complains Bankman-Fried.

"Your brows are a dead giveaway," replies Sheehan.

A tailor puts his sign on the door and signals Bankman-Fried to enter. The tailor throws unwashed T-shirt, cargo shorts, worn-out socks, rotting sneakers, and smelly underwear into a plastic garbage bag. Bankman-Fried returns to the bar. Whiffed with Dior Sauvage, he looks like a software engineer on his first day of work at Google—blue Oxford button-down collar, pressed chinos, new Sperry sneakers.

"Now get rid of your hyphenated last name," orders Sheehan. A distinguished gray-haired man in a pinstripe suit hangs his sign: Attorney-at-Law. Sam Bankman-Fried follows him through the door and emerges 20 minutes later as Mike Cameron.

Cameron returns to his barstool and finds Sheehan placing a 16-ounce ball-peen hammer on a cutting board atop the bar. "Put your laptop and phone here on the board," Sheehan commands. Cameron meekly complies. The bartender, now with protective goggles, raises the hammer and smashes both computing appliances to smithereens.

"May I have a cup of coffee?" asks Cameron. He balances the coffee on his right knee, which immediately begins to "jackhammer up and down at roughly four beats per second," as graphically described in *Going Infinite* by Michael Lewis. "2 ... 1 ... 0—Liftoff!" Coffee and cup leave the launchpad, ricochet off the fan, and shatter on the beamed ceiling, raining coffee drops and porcelain chips.

Sheehan looks up: "Have to work on the jackhammer. Traces of Bankman-Fried still there."

Neighbors 1943 and 2023
1943

On a chilly April afternoon Mr. Murphy crosses the street, passes the playpen under the elm tree, and notes Don holding the railing, standing, laughing, and shivering. He climbs Rosemary's steps and knocks on her door. She opens the door: "What is it, Mr. Murphy?"

"Your baby in the playpen is cold."

2023

My neighbor knocks frantically on the front door. Strange. In spite of living here for 30 years, I have never met her and don't know her name.

"Come out," she pleads.

Suspicious, I switch from RING to camera #2 over the garage. A fluffy grey Persian longhair is sleeping on the driveway, one eye open.

The back door starts creaking. I switch to camera #3. A large green bullfrog is in my rose garden, croaking.

I switch back to RING. "May I offer you coffee or moringa hot tea?" I ask.

"Neither, thank you. I just shot my husband."

"Is he still moving?"

"I think so."

"You might prefer a dram of Old Bushmills, then."

"Yes, that does sound better."

"I'll pass it through the mail slot."

Lolo's Recipe

Microwave steamed corn
cooked with my grandchild.
Lolo in kitchen
two at the table.
Unshucked corn on board
large knife from the rack
remove tip and stem
my cut first, then theirs.
Time set two-forty
tongs steady in hand
cold water bathes ears
stripping husks and silks.
Corn dried on towel
then placed on the plate
eyes closed as we taste
fresh love on the cob.

Sleepless Night Sounds

Magda snores lightly
Deep breaths and faint snorts.
My cancer cough calls
I wait for my next.
Silence a moment
Before snores resume.
Lupita asleep
Her crib at our side
Two-year granddaughter
Laughs loud in her sleep.
Joy bubbles over
From sleep into dreams.
Rain patters on panes
Thunder barks and fades
Breeze jingles the blinds.
I glance at the ceiling
And see dawn's greeting
I'm still alive.

The Odd Couple

By 2023, my OLLI in-person classes—creative writing and Improv 101—had begun to free me from my COVID-19 pandemic loneliness. I had new friends, and my few social skills were working better. Restored human connection brought a dormant quest to the surface, a search for new adventure and challenge. By luck, my Improv 101 instructor decided to teach a six-week acting class, called *Let's Put on a Play*.

Despite years of playing roles that the stage of life requires, I had never acted in theater or received acting instructions. The prospect of starting from zero scared and attracted me. To my happy surprise, two of my classmates were also octogenarians who had no prior experience in theater. I had met both in Improv 101: Sheila Goodman, bubbling with a delightful, uninhibited sense of humor, and Jack Christie, a retired proctologist. You read that correctly. We soon realized that we shared two characteristics that would bind and haunt us throughout this new adventure.

First, we each had a deep but different sense of humor. Second, we were intimidated by entering the kindergarten of theater in our ninth decade. Would memory, voice, mannerisms, balance, and ability to follow instructions in a new language be there to help us?

***

We were reassured by our teacher, Randy Letzler, who became The Director. Her career in New York theater, television, and teaching gave her the ability to detect our insecurities and strengths and to communicate skills that dampen the former and enhance the latter. The purpose of her acting class, like that of her Improv 101, was for us to have fun.

Sheila and I were given roles in a 15-minute segment from Neil Simon's *The Odd Couple*. I was Felix Unger; Sheila was Cecily Pigeon. Or was it, Gwendolyn Pigeon?

Jack was assigned the role of Bruce Wayne (Batman) in *Clark and Bruce*, a 15-minute one-act play about the two superheroes, now retired.

Because Sheila and I rehearsed together, I was better acquainted with our problems. At the first few rehearsals, Sheila couldn't remember a single line, and she often had trouble reading one. Insurmountable disadvantages? Not on your life. Her exuberant wit, quick mind, and instant repartee made her a natural master of the *ad lib*. Through the weeks of rehearsal, she received many tips for memorizing the script. Fortunately, none worked. She was always perfectly in character, and we fellow cast members happily adjusted to her lines as they were either read or invented.

I was the haunted one. After recording the lines of the other characters in *The Odd Couple*, leaving blank spaces for my Felix, I downloaded the recording to my computer.

Naturally, the suggestion for this exercise came from The Director. Every day, I would rehearse with my computer. Once a week, I tested the result at class rehearsal. I was terrible. So bad at memorizing my lines that at the next-to-last rehearsal, Randy insisted that I read and forget memorizing. I was not having fun. I had transferred my lifelong OCD tendencies, which had served me well as a surgeon, to memorizing a script. Practice and more practice were supposed to yield a perfect result.

I had repressed the results of psychological testing six years before. Not being able to memorize this simple, brief script was the first overt sign of my dementia. The Director and my three fellow cast members in *The Odd Couple* witnessed its public unveiling. I came out of the closet and began to share my vulnerability—in speaking with classmates and writing my memoir.

Jack had a lack of confidence about memorizing the script similar to mine, but he was more flexible about reading lines. His OCD tendencies were better focused. An advantage of proctology over ophthalmology?

Our command performance took place in the largest classroom of Founders Hall to a packed audience of eighty. I did okay without reading my lines, perhaps by incorporating Sheila's tactics.

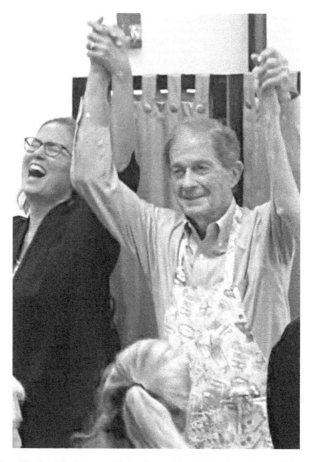

Fig. 45. 2023. Don as Felix from *The Odd Couple* and Gwen Schooler from *Basket Case* in the group curtain call after the performances in *Let's Put on a Play*.

Chapter 24

Genes and a Serial Killer

Serious problems can lurk in the caves and tunnels of our genetic histories, whether or not we are aware in advance. One of ours was a serial killer.

Our daughter-in-law, Tiffany, was a 35-year-old brunette, green-eyed mother of three: 12-year-old daughter Nina, seven-year-old son Ezra, and two-year-old daughter Lupe.

Tiffany had graduated from Temple Law School seven years before. She had walked proudly across the stage at graduation to a standing ovation from other graduates, holding newborn Ezra in her arms and the hand of toddler Nina, receiving her diploma and looking forward to a bright future.

Tiffany's maternal grandmother had died from pancreatic cancer at age 76 soon after diagnosis, without receiving treatment. A serial killer had stolen into Tiffany's home. Ten percent of pancreatic cancer cases are hereditary.

In February, 2023, Tiffany suddenly suffered severe back pain, which radiated to both sides. A CT scan showed a cyst of the pancreas, with carcinoma a leading probable cause.

Although the pain disappeared completely within two days, the CT findings were worrisome. Within two weeks, an endoscopic biopsy of the cyst yielded thick mucinous contents but no cellular material for histopathologic diagnosis. She consulted pancreatic cancer surgeons near home at the Hospital of the University of Pennsylvania and Jefferson Hospital in Philadelphia. After these consultations and the surgical procedure, Tiffany and her husband, my son Keith, called for my advice. As a Johns Hopkins School of Medicine graduate, they knew my bias. I arranged for Tiffany to receive a third opinion from the Skip Viragh Multidisciplinary Pancreatic Cyst Clinic at Hopkins. She and Keith asked me to accompany them. I would be an informed extra set of ears and a loving parent.

Tiffany's appointment was with Dr. William Burns, an affable surgeon with an impeccable background. Dr. Burns had thoroughly reviewed her history, tests, radiographic studies, and the opinions of the previous consultants before she arrived. He listened carefully as Tiffany told her story.

He asked a few questions, taking his time. His extensive experience gave reassuring answers.

"You have a rare type of pancreatic tumor we see most frequently in young women, probably no more than one percent of all pancreatic cancers. This colloid carcinoma, or papillary mucinous neoplasm, is first detected as a cyst of the pancreas, often as an incidental finding. In your case, a coincidence unrelated to your abdominal pain. The cyst can remain benign for years but usually progresses to the malignant stage."

"Is that why my cyst had only mucinous contents on biopsy and no cells?" asked Tiffany.

"Exactly," said Dr. Burns. "This gelatinous substance is one of the characteristics that gives me confidence to put this diagnosis before other possibilities in your case. It also makes me think that less radical surgery and a better chance of success might be possible for you."

After discussing the mechanics of surgery at Hopkins and his experience with the Philadelphia centers, we shook hands and left for our car. By chance he was waiting for our same elevator.

"Is there a restaurant you recommend for lunch within walking distance?" asked Keith.

"Helmand Kabobi on Wolfe Street," he said without hesitation, "a great Afghan place near Welch Library."

We were changed people when we arrived at the restaurant—no longer the worried three miracle seekers who had arrived at Dr. Burns's office that morning. Tiffany now had concrete information to finalize the decision she had already been working toward.

Our lunch conversation debated the relative merits of *shorwa*, vegetarian *aush*, and *banjan borani*. We agreed that the cardamom hot tea was the best we'd ever tasted. No one discussed pancreatic cancer.

We left Helmand Kabobi leaning into a typical windy 57-degree gray May day and stopped at the corner of Wolfe and Monument Streets before walking west to the parking garage. I couldn't resist giving a brief Hopkins walking tour: "Across Monument Street was the entrance to the Women's Clinic building during the 1960s. Next door, to the south on Wolfe Street, was the pick-up bay for the morgue at the pathology building. Here is the place where I saw a mother in a wheelchair holding her newborn baby as she was wheeled from the obstetrics unit of Women's Clinic to her husband's waiting car. At the same time, a funeral van was backing to the pick-up bay to collect a dead body."

"Birth, life, and death at a glance," Keith deadpanned.

"You've heard the story before?"

"Ever since birth."

Chapter 25

Death of My Parents

Bus Stop, Stuffed Tomatoes, and an Iguana

I was fortunate to have lived long enough to help ease both parents' departures from life. Maybe you will also have the chance to make things easier for your parents at the end.

My dad's memory died when he was in his late seventies. By the time Mom, Janet, and I realized that he had Alzheimer disease, he couldn't remember what he had eaten for breakfast, whose house he was in, or his best friend's name. I could never again have a conversation with him.

Although the experience is at times difficult for caregivers, the three of us agreed that no one had ever lived a happier last 10 years of life than Dad. As Richard Ford says in *Be Mine*: "It's widely acknowledged that people live longer and stay happier the more stuff they can forget or ignore."

Dad did have a few months of strange behavior and transient anger without violence. He escaped to the Cadillac dealership to buy a new car and was angry at Mom when she caught him and returned the car. Dad had a wandering phase, escaping to stroll in his pajamas. Mom slept on the entryway floor to prevent him from leaving at night. When I next visited, I installed a childproof latch high inside the front door. She then returned to sleep with him in their bedroom.

Dad settled into a contented routine. He would look out the living room window for hours, explaining to me that he was waiting for the bus so he could go play baseball with his friends. Helping wash, dry, and fold laundry in the condo basement was a two-hour exercise that brought him smiles and a nap when Keith and I visited.

I called Dad's contented routine, the "Bus Stop" stage of his dementia. Memory had diminished enough to shield him from the frustration of facing how much he had lost. My caregiver task at this stage was to sit with him, listen to his stories without judgment, without inquiring who his friends were, or where the baseball field was. I needed to accept his dreams, fantasies, and fragmented memories without question.

After my own two series of psychological tests for Alzheimer Disease in 2014 and 2016, each lasting for two days, I decided to monitor my own condition. I would not return once a year to suffer through masochistic days of tests that magnify mental images of my failure to remember a list of words or reproduce a few simple geometric shapes. Both tests, two years apart, had been glaring, humiliating reminders of what I had lost. The "Stuffed Tomato" stage precedes the "Bus Stop" stage and is more threatening because memory can still test reality.

I recognized the "Stuffed Tomato" stage one evening when Dax's wife, Marion, prepared her deceased mother's favorite meal—stuffed tomatoes. Only Kai, my grandson, and I were at the table. Marion brought to the table a hot casserole dish from the oven with four tomatoes stuffed with seasoned ground beef and a serving spoon about three inches in diameter. The stuffed tomatoes were each five inches in diameter. I started to serve the stuffed tomatoes while Marion and Magda were still working behind the kitchen counter.

I balanced the first stuffed tomato on the serving spoon. It wobbled precariously as I lifted it from the hot casserole dish toward the plate. Magda saw the impending disaster and hurried from behind the counter to snatch the serving spoon. I growled, "I can do this," and dumped the stuffed tomato onto the plate.

My memory, eight years after my initial diagnosis, was better than Dad's after a similar period. Details of my career as an eye surgeon were not the images I saw as I juggled the stuffed tomato, but they were close enough to remind me of what I had lost.

What should be the caregiver's response in the "Stuffed Tomato" stage of dementia?

Distraction, of course.

Instead of scurrying from behind the kitchen counter to snatch the serving spoon, Magda could have looked up to the ceiling and called to me from behind the counter, "Don, there's an iguana on the chandelier!" The "iguana dementia distraction" would have let me drop the stuffed tomato onto the casserole dish, look up to the chandelier, and avert a moment of anger. While I was scanning the chandelier, Magda could have cut the stuffed tomato into quadrants and served them safely onto the plate.

The Improv Theory of Memory Retrieval

Part I: My Comedy Career

"My favorite comedian on Planet earth" – Stephen Colbert

"The funniest woman in the world" – Judd Apatow

These two American comedy icons are referring to Maria Bamford.[9] Since you are my improv confidants, I'm going to let you in on a show business secret. I opened for Maria Bamford in 2011.

---

9. Maria Bamford, *Sure, I'll Join Your Cult: A Memoir of Mental Illness and the Quest to Belong Anywhere.* New York: Simon & Schuster, 2023.

In order to project a low profile and facilitate crowd control, the comedy show was advertised as a reunion of 1966 graduates of the Johns Hopkins School of Medicine. One year before the show, Dr. Diane Becker asked me to be MC. I spent the year compiling a voluminous collection of biographical detail, photographs, and gossip on all members of the class of 1966. I organized the material into a world-class 45-minute PowerPoint presentation. The evening before the meeting Diane called with one last change: "Don, we've also invited the daughter of one of your classmates to the event. I'll introduce her after your presentation."

"Fine," I said. These affairs always involve some last-minute adjustments, so I didn't ask for details.

The next evening, in the auditorium packed with M.D. '66 graduates, friends, and family, I droned on for 45 minutes with illustrated biographical details of my classmates' achievements and quirks.

After polite applause, Diane took the microphone: "It gives me great pleasure to introduce the daughter of one of your classmates, Joel Bamford, and his lovely wife, Marilyn. Their daughter, Maria, lives in Los Angeles, has starred in film, TV, audio, and video recordings, and toured the country with her delightful, famously bizarre vignettes. Here is Maria Bamford!"

Part II: Memory Reorganization and Reassembly

An email from a classmate, Lew Becker, set me straight. Lew had notes, recordings, and photos of all our medical school class reunions. He wrote that Maria's performance was at our 2007 reunion. My PowerPoint presentation as MC was at our 2011 reunion, four years later! In 2023 I had reassembled memories incorrectly to form an entirely new and different story. The switch raises a question that I had never considered. My fragmented memories from 10 and 16 years before behaved like packets or particles, not clouds. I could not recall all of the 2007 meeting, nor all of the 2011 meeting. I could not remember either story in its entirety. I selected fragments from each to construct a new, more enjoyable story.

Unfortunately, in the process of discovering what had actually happened, I lost my comedy career. I never opened for Maria Bamford.

Perhaps our concept of retrieval, the third memory process, is an oversimplification. Reorganization, reassembly, and a touch if imagination may also be involved—the improv theory of memory retrieval. It might explain how Dad stayed so relaxed while waiting for the bus to play baseball with his friends.

Crossing the River

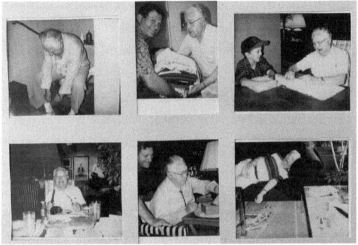

Fig. 46. Memphis, 1999. *"A Day in the Life of Daddy Nick"*
by Keith Nicholson.

Dad dearly loved Gloria Billingsly, his daytime caregiver, and eagerly awaited her arrival: "Gloria gives the best baths in the world," he explained. She would occasionally take him to her home for the day to nap in her husband Maurice's recliner chair.

The same Christmas card would greet him every morning on the breakfast table: "Robert sent a Christmas card! Let's read his note. He is so sweet."

I became manager of caregivers. Each month I flew to Memphis with my copy of *The 36-Hour Day* and a spreadsheet of short-term goals, doctors' appointments, adult daycare arrangements, and how to keep dear Gloria happy.

Our proudest achievement was for Mom and Dad to continue living together in their own home until the end of his life, nine years after diagnosis.

Mom lived for 10 years after Dad died—socially engaged, eager learner, and popular speaker at public book reviews. Her lifelong speaking and debating skills, evident even at age 90 in our interviews, would have made her a star in Lucia Small's *Girl Talk*.

We were once watching the sun set over the Memphis Pyramid when Mom taught me about the earth's axis of rotation. She brought a contractor's protractor to her eighth-floor west side window. Using the tree line as the horizontal base, she traced the setting sun from above the pyramid to the horizontal line. The angle of descent was 23.5° from vertical. "That's because the earth's axis is 23.5° from the plane of earth's orbit around the sun," she explained.

I was 65 years old.

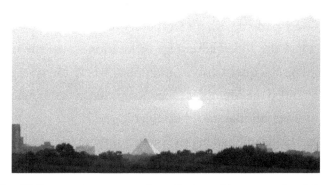

Fig. 47. Sunset view to west from Parkway House condominium.

I continued my monthly visits to Memphis to manage her finances and give Janet a break from errands and doctors' appointments.

Each month Mom and I would also have fun—concert, theater, or musical tickets, dinners prepared for neighborhood widow friends, new restaurants and our old reliable—Anderton's Oyster Bar.

I took her on road trips, like those our family had enjoyed in the 1950s. We drove with a friend to Hot Springs for a long weekend and, by ourselves another time, to Cape Girardeau to see their lifelong friend, Jack Fleming, at a nursing home.

In October, 1999, Mom left Dad in the Bright Glade Health and Rehabilitation Center in Memphis, so that she, Janet, Robert, and I could attend Trip and Stacey's wedding in Michigan. The staff and the facility at Bright Glade seemed first class and were highly recommended. Mother and the rest of us were pleased with his temporary home.

It had the added advantage of location across the street from The Racquet Club of Memphis, where for years Dad had attended the Memphis Open tennis tournament, with its cast of international stars. He felt at home.

In Michigan I had my last opportunity to spend a happy, joking week with Robert.

At the wedding reception dinner, I broke a personal wedding tradition and told the guests: "I'm not giving Trip and Stacey the Traditional Wedding Carrots I gave Robert and Janet. Instead, I've brought a mesh bag, like those for lemons in grocery produce departments. It contains pieces of used soap bars. Mother attaches one of these soap bags to the kitchen faucet to wash her hands. This is the perfect 'Stay Frugal Like Mama Nick' gift for this young couple."

Robert stood and shot back, "I know why you abandoned the Traditional Wedding Carrots. You are so old that you don't even remember what that meant!"

We returned from the wedding October 10, Mom and Janet to Memphis, Robert to Tulsa, and I to Miami. Mom soon noticed that Dad wasn't as active as before, couldn't be led to walk, and preferred to stay in bed.

He died quietly October 19 at Bright Glade. I should have reviewed his list of medications from the first day. Hospices and nursing homes often give sedatives to patients who can't tolerate them.

Dad was cremated, and Mom kept his ashes in the trunk of her car for a couple of years. Her frugality lived beyond the grave. She had me find the two charred metal hip prostheses in Dad's box of ashes, wash them, and accompany her to the Campbell Clinic. There she asked Dr. Knight if he could use them on a different patient. "No, thank you, Mrs. Nicholson," smiled the orthopedic surgeon, "I now use a newer model." A few months later, she said it would be a good time for her, Janet, and me to scatter his ashes over Robert's grave, near Millington.

Our memories of deceased loved ones are often crowded into the corner of the lives they occupied during the period leading to their death—weeks, months, or even years. For several years, Dad's Alzheimer decade replaced the rest of his life in my memory. That wasn't fair to him. Writing this memoir has brought back more of the life he shared with me. Family road trips, teaching me to drive, gently coaxing—never demanding—that I accompany him to learn golf and tennis, teaching me in his own peculiar way about the birds and bees, hosting my teenage birthday parties in the screening room, retrieving me and my friends from the Jackson County Jail, planting the dream of attending Stanford, celebrating graduations, marriages, births.

Even in his Alzheimer decade, his love and humor continued to brighten my life.

Mother concealed her approach to death so well that only in retrospect do I understand what was happening.

One time we had talked briefly about old age. She summed it up as follows: "Your sixties are your young old age. You feel well, can do anything, and live happily with your spouse. Your seventies are years of plain old age. Your eighties are the years of old, old age—everything is harder. Your nineties can best be discarded." She died at age 94. I imagine she felt that it was time to go. She had already lived too many years in the decade that "best be discarded."

After Dad's death, Janet helped Mom sell the Parkway House condominium and find a two-bedroom apartment in an assisted living complex near the University of Memphis. I continued to visit once a month and planned our evenings as before, season tickets to Playhouse on the Square, concerts, dinner with a friend in her new apartment. The second bedroom gave me a place to sleep. In fact, in her first year lease Mom had negotiated a monthly rent equal to that of a one-bedroom apartment!

Her new location was on a different 10-mile course for my morning run—through the center of the University of

Memphis campus, past the Japanese cherry trees and Memphis Botanic Garden on Cherry Road, then across the Audubon golf course, one of the places where Dad and I played on Saturdays.

A year before she died, Mom began to slow down. She had no complaints, including pain. She did have less appetite, even for the special dinners I knew she liked; earlier bedtimes; and more sleepless nights.

One afternoon in March, 2011, Janet's husband, Larry, was making his weekly wellness rounds to Mom's apartment. He knocked. No answer. He knocked loudly and called, "Rosemary ... Rosemary." No answer. Management opened the door, and they found Mom moaning in pain on the floor, unable to stand. Janet came immediately.

The ambulance took her to the hospital emergency room. There began a series of examinations and tests that lasted the whole night. Janet, an R.N., begged for something to relieve the pain, which continued to double Mom up. "Not until we have the test results," called the ER nurse over her shoulder.

More hours, more writhing, more agony. Larry's son, Stephen, had by then arrived, and the three spent the night taking turns holding Mom's hand and trying to give comfort in an intolerable situation. I was on a plane from Miami to Memphis that wouldn't arrive until mid-morning.

About dawn, all tests, including a CT scan, were complete. The scan showed disseminated metastatic carcinoma throughout her lungs, abdomen, and pelvis. At Janet's insistence, the nurse finally gave an injection of morphine. Mom was still grimacing and crying a half-hour later, so Janet asked for another dose. Half was given.

Mom relaxed and smiled. The morphine had let her feel calm enough to die.

The CT scan told me what the past year of gradual, uncomplaining deterioration had been. While the undetected cancer had been filling her body with malignant cells, diminishing her appetite and strength, increasing her pain, she had been protecting her family from knowing what she was going through. It was pure stoicism.

The corner of Mom's life that occupied my memory for 10 years after her death was my failure and her lingering agony. Finally, when I wrote the notes of our 2005 conversations into the story, reality hit home. This ending was how she had lived her life. She overcame seeing her abusive, alcoholic father put a knife to her mother's throat in public. She lived through watching him choke her mother's breath until she fainted. She listened and obeyed her father when he told her, "If you don't accept the drama scholarship for college and stay home with me, I can fix my alcohol problem." She spent nights in the sleeping porch bed with him. We'll never know the limits of his abuse. My mother shared her stories with me in a kind of code, never in explicit detail.

Stoicism let her love shine. We kidded her for years about her sense of denial. As captured in one of our interviews, she joined in: "Alzheimer for him and denial for me. That was a good combination."

In retrospect I think that denial was one of several traits that helped her through difficult times. My memory of her will not be the last corner of her life, a year of decline and death. It will be Mom carrying two pillows and a blanket across a darkened living room to my father, collapsed on the floor, unable to rise or be lifted. She covers him with the blanket, places the two pillows, and cuddles at his side, "So he won't be afraid if he wakes up."

Chapter 26

My Memoir Revision

Through the haze of receding sleep I see Magda sitting at my bedside.

"Don, you're dying."

With IV, nasal oxygen, and urinary catheter working full time, I wheeze, "Why are you telling me?"

"I have to remind you."

"Why?"

"Well, it's your cancer ..."

"I know *how I'm dying* ..." I take a breath. "Why do you have to remind me *that I am dying*?"

"Your dementia needs my help. For example, you never remembered that you didn't get it up on our wedding night."

"I don't need to remember ... You have reminded me every week for forty-five years."

"And the Peruvian woman I uncovered by finding a receipt in your wallet."

"She was Ecuadorian."

"You spent three weeks recovering from Hurricane Dennis in bed with the neighbor?"

"Medical practice taught me ... good rest with a soft pillow stimulates recovery."

"Your memoir is about a Boy Scout, not the atrocious person you are."

"My memoir means my memories about my life."

A nurse with a syringe knocks and enters the room. "Time for your morphine," she sings.

"I'll wait outside," Magda tells her.

"How are you this morning, Dr. Nicholson?"

"About the same, Grace. Can you please give me a double? Better, a triple?"

"We have this discussion every day, and you know the answer: NO!"

"I have a hundred dollars tucked away for you," I beg. "I'm desperate."

"I'm giving you the dose the doctor ordered. Rules are rules."

She injects the morphine slowly through an injection port of the IV tube.

Entering the room, Magda smiles at Grace and returns to her armchair.

"About your memoir. I hired your previous editor to help me write a more honest version. She already knows your sanitized version, so this shouldn't take more than a few weeks.

"Here is a list of chapters I've given her to add: incest, impotence, intemperance, infidelity, pregnancy, paternity, abortion, disability, STIs, child neglect, ectopic pregnancy and forced menopause. I'll dictate the details for each chapter. The editor will transcribe and edit the manuscript."

"Ectopic pregnancy and forced menopause?"

"The time you aimed your sperm at my cervix and caused a cervical ectopic pregnancy. The emergency hysterectomy left me in menopause for the last forty years."

"I aimed my sperm and hit your cervix? ... Maybe, instead of squeezing, I jerked the trigger."

Magda lowers her voice. "I can't discuss the worst."

"'Z's conviction and prison sentence?"

"Yes."

"You're right to leave that out. "Z" suffered enough."

This was a good last conversation—humor and sympathy.

***

A driver sat me on the back of his tiny motorbike, and we headed for the edge of the desert. Every so often we saw a pipe extending upward from ground level six or eight feet, usually leaning a few inches from vertical. The pipes each emitted a faint orange-yellow flame, which gave little light, but thick smoke and strong acrid odor. "Flammable gas from underlying waste deposits?" I wondered. Passing dry desert brush and prickly pear cactus, we headed toward the ocean as dusk descended. In a concealed dry arroyo the driver hid the motorbike for his return trip, and we walked west on the path. Other hikers walked past us in silence, also headed west. An attractive alto, singing a familiar song, smiled as she passed.

Ahead we spied a cluster of the pipes, each tipped by a lance of orange-yellow smoky flame. Twenty figures gathered near the pipes. A celebration? Approaching closer, we could see a half-dozen wooden platforms lying flat on the rocky ground. Each platform was roughly square, measured 10 feet or less on each side and six inches elevated from the ground. One or two people stood or sat on each stage, speaking in normal tones. We circulated in small groups, listening to the actors discuss serious matters—birth of a deformed baby, diminishing population, a shrinking oasis. We approached one stage with a lone woman at its center, the singer who had passed us on the trail. She smiled, then gasped a silent scream, clenched her fist to her chest, and fell face down on the stage. Suspecting a heart attack, I rushed to the stage, rolled her over onto her back, and checked carotid pulse and breath sounds. None of either. I shouted, hoping for her response. Nothing. I knelt in the familiar resuscitation position, arms down, elbows locked, heel of my open right hand on her sternum, heel of the left on top of the right. I began to pump and relax, increasing the rate. The heel of my bottom hand suddenly struck the wooden stage—THUD—THUD. She had disappeared. The four spectators clapped silently, then dispersed to other stages. I stepped back to the ground, and we resumed our stroll to the ocean.

The next morning I died in my sleep. Magda was dictating her first new chapter for my memoir revision.

My Legacy

My legacy is a memorial to my parents, the **Howard and Rosemary Nicholson Scholarship** fund, which I endowed at the Johns Hopkins School of Medicine Development Office, 750 E. Pratt St., Baltimore, MD 21202. Your contributions are appreciated and tax-deductible.

In the 10 years since I endowed the fund for students who, like me, were the first in their families to graduate from college, 10 deserving students have received financial aid—one each from Colombia, Haiti, Brazil, and Ethiopia, the rest from the United States.

My parents' love still lives.

Scattergun Memoir Technique

How many of you would like to leave memories of your lifetime to your grandchildren?

This appendix tells how I wrote mine.

I.   Shoot.

A scattergun spreads small projectiles across a wide area. A memoir scattergun patterns those projectiles horizontally, along a timeline—the span of your life.

II.   Begin writing.

Each mark in the target is a memory. Examine one point and write about it. Relax. If no new thoughts come, pick another point, examine it, and write the memory it contains. This process leaves a series of disconnected memories, which may disappoint you. Don't worry. Keep repeating. One day, your just-written memory will release a new, unexpected visitor, as if she had been hiding nearby—a new memory. She begs you to write her story and include her in your book.

A creative writing course at this stage may help you.

III.   Organize.

Ugh.

You have a thousand memories, most of which remain scattered along the span of your life, a hundred that have magically connected to a nearby memory. Sit and review. Put them in order, either by the period of your life when they occur, or by association with other memories, later or earlier. Now you have a semi-outline. But you have only 20,000 words, and your editor has told you that a book requires twice that number.

IV.   Take a deep breath.

There are other stories in your life that you haven't tapped. Your father died, but your mother is still alive. Buy a digital voice recorder, or use your smartphone voice recording app, practice a while, then interview your mother. She should be comfortable, perhaps seated at her own dining room table. You should also be comfortable, perhaps wearing your sandals. Keep the interview sessions short—one hour is perfect, maybe a total of four one-hour sessions altogether. Be sure to dedicate one session to her memories of her deceased husband, your father. If he is still alive, instead, set up a separate series of interviews with him.

V.   Transcribe the interviews.

Many online firms can prepare accurate typed transcriptions from your interviews. I sent files of my four one-hour interviews 17 years after I recorded them. They arrived from transcriptionpuppy.com within 48 hours and were done perfectly. These companies usually work with lawyers on depositions and probably like to receive a loving conversation between daughter or son and mother.

VI.   Edit and abridge the transcription.

You never thought anyone would say "just" or "and", or "maybe" so many times during a cherished, meaningful conversation.

Do the editing yourself. No one else could appreciate and correct its nuances.

The next part is fun. Spoken conversations are not good prose. You need to review and improve the transcript at least as many times as you would a first draft. Editing should reduce the length of your transcript by at least 10 percent.

VII.   Incorporate the edited conversations into your manuscript for the book.

I used "My Mother's Life" as a separate chapter for her four interviews, inserted just before "Retirement." Reviewing and editing the written transcription gave me a new, beautiful view of my mother's love that I had never appreciated, even though I had listened to our recorded interviews many times during the years between our conversations and the transcription and editing. If you are fortunate enough to have interviews with your father, transcribe and edit his interviews to include in his chapter "My Father's Life."

VIII.   Illustrations.

During your lifetime you have collected albums, scrapbooks, shoeboxes, and computer files filled with thousands of photographs of you and your family. Select 50 or fewer that illustrate key moments and people in your life. All can be edited and digitized to prepare for publication. Write the legend for each photograph.

IX.   Word count.

Now you can see the numerical effect of your added, edited interview and illustrations.

XI.   Flesh it out.

Memories beget memories, creating a treasure vault you can visit often. Among the memories you have already recorded, you will find others waiting to appear. Add Contents, List of Illustrations, References, Appendix, and Acknowledgements. You have arrived.

About the Author

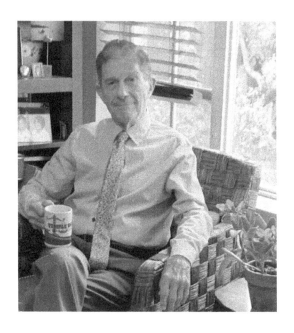

Don Nicholson, M.D., is a graduate of the Johns Hopkins University School of Medicine and a retired professor who had been an ambassador of ophthalmology and educator to specialists in Latin America, the Caribbean, and Spain.

When Nicholson was 74 years old, the chief of geriatric memory at the University of Miami medical school concluded after thorough testing that he had Alzheimer disease, which had also affected his father. *My Dementia Defense* is a multifaceted memoir he began during the COVID-19 pandemic. More than jotting a few memories for his grandchildren, writing the book became his defense against progression of dementia.

Printed in the USA
CPSIA information can be obtained
at www.ICGtesting.com
LVHW010537140624
783163LV00002B/4